# Clinical Report of Paida Lajin on Thyroid Disease

Hongchi Xiao

2022

A Clinical Report of PaidaLajin on Thyroid Disease

by Hongchi Xiao

Copyright © 2024 Pailala Institute

All Rights Reserved

No part of this book may be reproduced or transmitted in any form or by any means, electronic or mechanical, including photocopying, recording, or by any information storage and retrieval system without written permission from the author, except for the inclusion of brief quotations in a review.

Pailala Institute

A nonprofit organization in California, USA

36 Ovation, Irvine

CA 92620, USA

Email: admin@pailala.org

Editors: Alice Fava, Ivor Noble

Manager: Shen Jun Zhi

ISBN: 9798326302496 (print)

First Edition Printed in the USA

# Dedication & Acknowledgement

This work is dedicated to my family, friends, volunteers, and team members who have been supportive all along, particularly during tough times, and to people across the world who are open to the idea of self-healing through Paida Lajin.

My special thanks to the following volunteers who helped me collecting, editing, compiling the cases in Chinese and translating them into English.

Chinese Team:

- Shen Jun Zhi
- Liu Ying
- Mo Fei

English Team:

- Ivor Noble
- Alice Fava

I also like to express my gratitude to all the teachers who taught me about Traditional Chinese Medicine, as well as the dedicated research done by Dr. Alfred Pischinger on matrix biology. Without them, I would not have recognized the power of self-healing through Paida Lajin or realized that Paida Lajin can be explained scientifically.

After so many years of hearing thousands of new testimonials and new cases that Paida Lajin has helped, I have recently come to realize that such an intricate design of the human body, and the gift of self- healing, can only be manifested by God. He continuously surprises me, giving me amazing insight into our world. Thank you, God.

# Medical Disclaimer

This book describes a self-healing practice, named as Paida Lajin with testimonials from its practitioners.

Paida Lajin is a self-healing exercise, including slapping and stretching, to improve the microcirculations of our body, so that our body can heal itself. Paida Lajin, by itself, does not treat or heal any illness.

Like yoga and t'ai chi, Paida Lajin is not a medical treatment, cannot replace medical treatment, nor has any conflict with any medication, because it does not use any medication or equipment. Anyone can try it.

The statements in this book have not been evaluated by the FDA. Self-healing with Paida Lajin is not intended to be a substitute for professional medical advice, diagnosis, or treatment. Always seek the advice of your physician or other qualified health care providers with any questions you may have regarding a medical condition. Never disregard professional medical advice or delay in seeking it because of the information provided herein.

This publication contains the opinions and witnesses of its author. It is intended to provide helpful and informative material on the subject covered.

The author and publisher specifically disclaim any responsibility for any liability, loss, or risk (personal or otherwise) incurred as a consequence, directly or indirectly, of the use and application of any of the contents of this book.

# Preface

In 2017, I was arrested and imprisoned. It was a turning point for Paida and Lajin self-healing method (hereinafter referred to as PL) and my life.

In the seven years before my incarceration, I had been traveling around the world to promote PL method by holding experience camps and lectures. During the seven years in prison, I have been researching and sorting out the clinical results of PL method. In short, I did clinical experiments for seven years and theoretical research for another seven years. Because of being in prison, I found myself becoming a scientific researcher. This is a title I never dreamed of. An American PL friend is a scientist. The therapeutic effect of just one tapping session exceeds the combined effects of all the treatments he tried over the years. So, he said to me, you are a scientist. I asked why. He said that the job of a scientist is nothing more than conducting experiments repeatedly in a certain way, and then summarizing and compiling the results to draw and then prove a new conclusion, and that is exactly what you are doing. The scientific experiments I did in the first seven years laid the foundation for the theoretical research of the next seven years. Specifically, medical experiments on human subjects are clinical experiments.

The main criticism of the PL method is that clinical experimentation does not confirm its authenticity and efficacy. However, the truth is exactly the opposite. For more than ten years, millions of people have done clinical experiments on themselves using PL, but no one has yet studied and compiled the results of these experiments! Although less than 1% of the PLA experimenters write reports on their clinical experiments, I collected thousands of real and vivid clinical reports. So my prison cell became the "Paida and Lajin Clinical Research Institute." Some people think that only experiments conducted by medical workers within the paradigm prescribed by medicine can be called clinical experiments. This is not true! Let us not confuse the form with the true purpose which is healing or freedom from disease. It is intellectually dishonest to do otherwise.

Regardless of whether drugs or methods are used for clinical trials, they are all purportedly undertaken to advance human health. In other words, the form and means all serve this goal. In the thousands of years of human medical history before the emergence of modern medicine, what we now call clinical experiments were simply implemented on the human body like the PL method. If it is just some kind of natural action, it will have no negative effects on the body. Even if herbal medicine is used, the negative effects will be far lower than the current chemical drugs. The key is whether these forms and means achieve their goals, that is, the efficacy. In other words, the true purpose (healing, freedom from disease) is more important than form. Besides, the PL method does not even use herbal medicine. It is simple to operate and low in cost, so the requirements for clinical trials are low. The only criterion is that the participant must be sick. In other words, anyone can participate in this experiment. From a medical perspective, this seems ludicrous. How can one method cure all diseases?

The truth is simple: if you find the common cause of all diseases and find a method to resolve this cause, you can naturally cure all diseases yourself with just one method. Is this possible? The only way to prove whether this is possible is through clinical trials. These thirty clinical reports summarize the efficacy of the PL method in self-healing hundreds of diseases. Because there are too many disease names, I can only briefly classify them according to people's common understanding, which may not necessarily conform to medical classification. Because people do not become ill according to medical and clinical standards, clinical trials of PL are more in line with human normality, that is, a person may suffer from multiple diseases more than ten or twenty. Since the PL method believes that all diseases are caused by blocked meridians, using the PL method to open up the meridians can self-cure many or even more than ten diseases at the same time. This is borne out in all my clinical reports. Because of this, some cases appear in different reports. The PL healing method aligns with human survival and ecological protection.

Western medicine clinical trials are almost always based on the effectiveness of a certain drug on a certain disease. That is, the drug has a clear target and generally has negative effects. Therefore, the experimental candidates and processes have to be strictly controlled. The PL method does not involve medication, nor does it set out to target specific illnesses. Instead, it targets the common cause of all

diseases-, blocked meridians. In the majority of cases, the result of unblocking the meridians is the self-healing of known and unknown illnesses. There is no need to use the method prescribed by Western medicine to perform the PL method. However, this does not mean rejecting Western medicine. Using Western medical instruments and standards to detect the clinical effects of PL is part of the clinical practice of PL, proving that PL and Western medicine can collaborate to learn from each other's strengths.

Some people will question the more than 90% efficacy of PL. That is understandable. We therefore welcome experts or anyone to criticize PL based on these results. But making rash comments without conducting clinical trials is not in keeping with the scientific spirit. I must emphasize here that no one method is suitable for everyone. Although this method is simple and effective, the human heart is extremely complex, the human subconscious is even more complex, and, as the body is a tool of the soul. The PL method cannot be suitable for everyone. To achieve complete healing, you need to combine PL with meditation and a spiritual practice .

Thirty clinical reports have been written so far, four of which have been translated into English and published: "Diabetes", "Hypertension", "Thyroid Disease", and "Pain and Depression". All proceeds from the publication of this series of books will be used for the public welfare promotion of PL and meditation practices. Since there are still more than 20 reports to be translated into English and published, we sincerely invite friends who understand English to join in translating the series of clinical reports on PL and promote PL and meditation to the world as soon as possible.

The series of PL reports that have been completed so far are as follows: "Clinical Report on Diabetes", " Clinical Report on Hypertension/Hypotension Paila ", "Clinical Report on Stroke", "Clinical Report on Kidney Disease", "Clinical Report on Pulmonary and Respiratory Diseases", " "Clinical Report on Gastroenterology", "Clinical Report on Dermatology", "Clinical Report on Gynecological Diseases", "Clinical Report on Depression and Mood Disorders", "Pain and Depression: Comparison of Clinical Cases between Western Medicine and Paila " , "Clinical Report on Thyroid Disease" "Clinical Report on Cancer and Tumors", "Clinical Report on Hepatobiliary Diseases", "Clinical Report on Neurodegenerative Diseases", "Clinical Report on Deafness and Tinnitus", "Clinical Report on Stomach Diseases", "Clinical Report on Pediatric Diseases", " "Clinical Report on Headache, Dizziness and Head Patting", "Clinical Report on Weight Loss, Beauty and Breast Enlargement", "Clinical Report on Femoral Head Necrosis, Ankylosis and Scoliosis", "Clinical Report on Sexual Function and Genitourinary System Disorders", "Clinical Report on Immune Function Diseases", "Clinical Report on Insomnia", "Clinical Report on Pain", "Clinical Report on Rheumatoid Arthritis and Fibromyalgia", "Clinical Report on Gout ", "Clinical Report on Varicose Veins, Phlebitis and Vasculitis" , "Heart disease clinical report", "Emergency clinical report", "Eye disease clinical report", "Toothache and oral disease clinical report", "Dark urine, brown urine (coffee urine), hematuria clinical report".

Finally, I would like to sincerely thank the Chinese and foreign volunteers who collected cases, printed, edited, and translated for the publication of this book!

——Xiao Hongci April 11, 2024

# Table of Contents

Dedication & Acknowledgement .................................................................. 3
Medical Disclaimer ........................................................................................ 4
Preface ............................................................................................................. 5
The Significance of the Clinical Report of Paida and Lajin ........... 12
Several terms concerning the Clinical Report of PL ....................... 32

    1. What is Paida and Lajin? ................................................................. 32

    2. What is Qi? What are meridians? ................................................. 33

    3. What are the HC? ........................................................................... 33

    4. What is Sha? .................................................................................... 44

    5. What are the main meridians in the human body? Where are they distributed in the body? ............................................................. 45

    6. What are the Universal Parts? ........................................................ 47

Introduction ................................................................................................ 48

Chapter 1 Statistical report of thyroid disease cases treated with PL .................................................................................................................. 50

    1. Overall results of PL: ....................................................................... 53

    2. The details of the various diseases are shown as below: ......... 53

    3.    Location and time of PL: ........................................................... 54

Chapter 2 Clinical Discussion of Thyroiditis, Hyperthyroidism, Hypothyroidism, and Thyroid Cancer ................................................. 56

    1-1 The self-healing path of chronic thyroiditis ............................ 56

    1-2 My hyperthyroidism and insomnia healed by PL .................. 59

    1-3 PL heals the eight-year hyperthyroidism and improves hot temper. ................................................................................................... 63

    1-4 Hyperthyroidism was healed and anxiety was significantly improved ................................................................................................ 65

    1-5 Hyperthyroidism antibodies were normalized by eight months of Lajin ..................................................................................... 65

1-6 Is Oedema all over the body only caused by the thyroid gland? .................................................................................................. 70

1-7 Therapeutic effect of high intraocular pressure and hyperthyroidism in an elderly German .......................................... 72

1-8 Daughter's thyroid antibodies were normalized after Paida .................................................................................................................. 74

1-9 Hyperthyroidism and lung nodules healed after six months of Paida ................................................................................................. 75

1-10 Verification with facts: Paida is very effective for hypothyroidism! ................................................................................. 81

1-11 Anterior heart pain, low white blood cells and hypothyroidism self-healed by stopping medication ................. 89

1-12 Constipation, weakness, frequent urination, low thyroid, and prostatitis ............................................................................... 94

1-13 Improvement of hypertension, heart disease, diabetes, and hypothyroidism after one year of PL ............................................ 97

1-14 Why did I stop all my medication? -- Thoughts about the first Anniversary of PL ...................................................................... 101

1-15 Effect of PL on hyperthyroidism, post-stroke ................. 115

1-16 Hyperthyroidism, Amenorrhoea, Constipation, Depression and Severe Weakness ...................................................................... 118

1-17 Severe hyperthyroidism, amenorrhea, depression and other 11 diseases healed by Paida .................................................. 122

1-18 Eight diseases of patient with hyperthyroidism healed by PL ............................................................................................................. 127

1-19 Hyperthyroidism, post-surgery symptoms, tumor indicators improved by Paida ........................................................ 133

1-20 Is her illness hyperthyroidism or heart disease? ............. 140

1-21 Hyperthyroidism sequelae and heart disease and cardiopathy ........................................................................................ 145

1-22 The sequelae of thyroid cancer self-heals ....................... 151

1-23 PL's recovery from thyroid cancer ..................................... 156

1-24 Mystery of HC from the sequelae of hyperthyroidism ...168

Chapter 3 Clinical discussion of goiter, nodule, tumor and cyst 177

2-1 Goiter cyst was healed by Paida of two elbows for 10 minutes .................................................................................. 177

2-2 Paida the thumb and fissure acupoint for two hours, thyroid nodules were healed ........................................................ 179

2-3 The size of thyroid nodule became negligible after two times of Paida ............................................................................ 181

2-4 How to Paida on the breast tumor and thyroid tumor? ...184

2-5 Thyroid and gynecological problems were all improved at physical examination after PL .................................................. 187

2-6 Thyroid surgery was canceled by 5 days of Paida .............. 197

2-7 My familial thyroid nodules are gone .................................. 199

2-8 My thyroid gland became smaller after Paida ..................... 201

2-9 The size of thyroid nodule had nearly gone after the fist Paida ........................................................................................... 208

2-10 Why can thyroid, pharyngitis and hepatitis B be self-healed? However, why are dizziness, insomnia and stomach problems persisting? ................................................................................. 214

2-11 Menopausal hot flashes, heartburn, insomnia, thyroid tumor and heart disease ........................................................... 220

2-12 Total improvement of dry syndrome, thyroid nodules, heart disease and depression ................................................... 227

2-13 A dozen diseases can be healed by PL ............................... 230

Appendix 1: Statistical Results of the Return Visits for the workshop ................................................................................... 239

Appendix 2: Statistical data analysis of PL (2018) ...................... 243

1. Gender ratio ....................................................................... 243

2. Overall efficiency of PL ..................................................... 243

3. Efficiency statistics for individual conditions ................. 243

4. Relation between the duration of PL and efficiency ...... 245

5. Relationship between PL and efficiency ..................246

6. Improvement effect of pain by PL ..........................247

Appendix 3: Statistics on the effect of PL self-healing method promoted by Boss Cao ..................................................249

Appendix 4: The statistics of 200 documented cases were promoted by Boss Cao ..................................................250

Appendix 5: Statistical results of Zhang Yumei PL Health Club in Huizhou, guangdong ..................................................252

Appendix 6: Investigation Report of PL by Hebei Zhao Ruihua ..................................................................................254

Appendix 7: Statistics on the effectiveness of the self-healing method of PL by Hubei Green Walnut ...........................259

Appendix 8: Shandong Yimu (retired driver) spread the effect of PL statistical table ..................................................261

# The Significance of the Clinical Report of Paida and Lajin

When we mention a clinical report, people just think that it will be the medical research report only prepared by doctors without knowing that the central concept of a clinic focuses on patients rather than doctors. In the Oxford Dictionary, the definition of clinical is "relating to the examination and treatment of patients and their illnesses, not theoretical research". Then the clinical experiment is to do experiments on patients by some methods, drugs, or instruments. Experiment with drugs or professional instruments can only undertaken by a doctor or a professional, because it involves certain dangers and professional skills. If it does not involve drugs or professional instruments, just non-medical body movements and methods, it is an experiment that everyone can do, such as, physical activities, yoga, aerobics and so on.

Paida and Lajin ("PL"), the two simple movements are simpler than physical activities, yoga, and aerobics because any common person only needs to spend a few minutes acquiring them. Hence, it is easier and more convenient to conduct experiments. If you fall ill, an experiment with PL becomes a clinical experiment, because you are treating the body and observing the results when you are practicing PL. Some people argue that the PL method is a lie. Doesn't it just give you an opportunity to do clinical trials? Just spend a week or a month experimenting with PL attentively, without spending a penny, you can reap the result naturally. Isn't it exactly what clinical trials are all about? There are a lot of scams in this world, but if you think it over, you will find that it is most difficult to cheat with a healing method. Because so long as you do the experiment, there will be only two results: effective or ineffective. The *Clinical Report of Paida and Lajin* is a summary and discussion of the clinical cases and sharing provided by the practitioners. The sources are all first-hand data of clinical experiments, so they are of great clinical value.

If you reflect on it more deeply, it will be easy for you to figure out that if only you are alive, you will use different methods to do clinical experiments. The most common method is to use all kinds of drugs and food. However, it is of greater risk with any method to take in something into the body. But people are quite willing to take the risk, so taking medicines is much more popular than PL. Some people take medicines just like having meals. They take drugs every day and several times a day. Some people even take drugs for years, more than a decade or even decades. You will be the lucky one if your health condition can be improved taking drugs! Because it is rare. Most of the clinical results of taking drugs are increasingly severe illnesses and increasing diseases. Instead of pressing a criticism on or a prejudice against it, I am telling you the facts. Meanwhile, it is a common phenomenon among all human beings. And this is also a clinical outcome.

In addition to oral medicine, there are also various clinical methods such as antibiotic injections, chemotherapy, radiotherapy, and surgery. If you want to ask about their clinical results, people who have done such clinical practice know clearly. Besides, there are various natural remedies, including Chinese herbal medicine and various external treatment methods. Any drug that enters the human body, even natural herbs, will have a negative effect. It is only less negative than chemical drugs. I am not showing my objection to using these common human clinical methods by listing them, but to illustrate that humans should use them with caution, that is to make maximum use of their strengths and minimize its negative effects. This is the meaning that I use "negative effects" rather than "side effects". It is to reduce harm to the human body.

No one can avoid doing clinical experiments with food, clothing, living and other lifestyles. For instance, if you take in excessive food, eat too much meat, drink devilishly, wear too little for beauty, stay up late for a long time, endure sleep debt and so on, you may cause harm to the body and fall ill. This is also the result of clinical experiments, which is of no difference from PL. It is somehow trying to process and observe your own body with a certain method. And your purpose is to feel better. But the interesting thing is that the clinical trials you do to feel better will make you feel worse. In other words, you get sick for that. But please do not forget that all the clinical experiments you do, namely the way you live, are determined by your mind.

We can see that disease is a decision that the mind made up using the body for this purpose. The disease derives from the heart exactly means the same. Lifestyle is a form of cardio-creation, while the more dominant way of cardio-creation is using negative emotions and false insights. Negative emotions are more apparent, but misconceptions, that is, wrong ideas and thoughts are invisible. Negative emotions are caused by false knowledge, so the two are the two sides of one coin, one inside and the other outside. But the misconception is more deeply hidden. The mind is different from the heart. It is shapeless and formless, so we can also call it spirit. Both negative emotions and misconceptions arise from the mind. The external event that causes emotions is the interpretation and illustration of the event by us. We interpret events according to our own ideas, that is, our thoughts, and then we have different emotions, because we all have different opinions. Hence, we can know that everyone is doing clinical experiments with their own thoughts and ideas, and the body has become a tool for the mind to do experiments. Then healing is not so much healing the body as correcting human knowledge.

Therefore, using PL to do clinical experiments is to use a new idea and a new way of thinking to deal with and observe the body, and to understand it with the mind. If it is of any difference from other natural methods, it is that it is more exciting to the mind and interacts more strongly with the heart, which can be said to point to the heart directly and change the heart. In other words, it causes more extensive and deeper heart disease and body disease, so the curative effect is more incredible. Many people who go deep and continue to do clinical practice with PL have to marvel at the miraculous effect of PL and call it a miracle. In fact, "Miracles are natural. When they do not occur something has gone wrong." (A Course in Miracles T-1.I.6) The magic effect of PL shows that this clinical experiment will restore the unnatural and distorted mind to normal, and some mistakes will be corrected, so the negative emotions are less, and the body controlled by the mind will return to normal. The changes in the body seem to be the improvement of biological indicators and physiological functions, which can be summarized into the more order and balance of the body energy field from a deeper level. In simple words  PL can be expressed as when the meridians are smoother, so people are healthier.

Why are so many people not able to understand PL? It is often because of the misunderstanding of the external characteristics of PL. So, it is easy for them to consider PL as the traditional therapy methods like scraping, cupping, acupuncture, massage, moxibustion and other external treatment, and ignore its huge impact and healing force in the spiritual level.

Any traditional external treatment method aims at getting through the meridians, promoting Qi and circulating blood. Therefore, a good curative effect will be reflected in the HC caused by the blockage. The stronger the activated Qi, the stronger and deeper the HC, the more diverse and lasting the ways of HC, the better the meridian clearing effect, and the better the effect of detoxification. Therefore, the key to read the clinical report is to see the state of HC, such as Sha, pain, itching, numbness, burping, farting, sweating, cold feeling, urine and feces, rash, vomiting, blisters, lumps, fatigue, coma and so on. Since HC is the process of turning out, resolve and discharge the disease with Qi, it indicates that the positive Qi and negative Qi are in a fierce game, so the original disease may be temporarily intensified, such as the original pain, blood pressure and blood sugar and other indicators as well as various discomfort, which just shows that the diagnosis and treatment are happening simultaneously. It is a good thing. But people who do not understand often fear and doubt, so they dare not to continue PL. The process and results of the clinical experiment just resolve this doubt.

Clinical results usually reveal that the more HC, the better the effect. But you can't see such various reactions of HC in other treatments. Some traditional Chinese medical doctors using Chinese medicine to treat patients may never encounter a HC, and even do not know what HC. Although some masters of traditional Chinese medicine know that HC is also called the Dizziness reactions, which is a strong kind of HC. It is rarely seen in clinical practice of general Chinese medicine. In the external treatment method, HC appears more often, but the degree and breadth are not enough, which is also one of the reasons for its limited curative effect. The most intuitive reason for the strong HC of PL is that its activated Qi is more intense, which can be said to be devastating and invincible. However, the most critical healing is that it is directed to the heart. The above-mentioned HC, although appearing on different parts of the body, work on the mind, the experiencer and the bearer. The mind feels and perceives the cause and result of disease in the HC and gradually changes.

The impact and healing of PL on the mind is comprehensive and multifaceted from beginning to end. When people are exposed to PL for the first time, their first reaction is mostly doubt. Can it be so simple, but with such a good curative effect? If we take a closer look, when they see the Sha that appears after Paida, and they think of the slapping they have experienced, they will immediately be frightened. With the deepening of clinical practice, there will be more unexpected HC, thus generating greater doubt and intense fear in them. In this process, many people will also face opposition and ridicule from the external world. Doubt and fear cause spiritual conflict prior to the start of PL or in its initial stage, which is the HC of heart disease. With the increasing and aggravating physical HC, each time, it may cause stronger HC to heart disease. If you get through these HC and reap a good effect, you will regard it as a treasure and be eager to spread it to relatives and friends, thinking that they will be as excited as you. But the result is often that you have to face more sarcasm. Especially amid the critical storm of rumors and media, your mind will encounter HC again. That is one of the reasons why many who enthusiastically promoted PL give up halfway after using PL to heal many chronic and stubborn diseases. More people stop PL or rarely practice PL after just getting better in the disease, because another bigger heart disease begins HC, that is, laziness.

Why are the HC to the heart disease caused by PL far more than other general external treatments?

That is because PL is a true self-healing method. Do you believe in PL? Do you apply PL? A what intensity? And for how long? What is the best method to overcome the physical and mental HC and so on? All this can only be decided by your mind. With other methods, including naturopathy, the decisions are made by others, and the donor and the recipient are separate. But the donor and the recipient PL is one. Even if you apply with each other or ask someone to help, you can only make decisions and choices on your own. It is also in this process that your knowledge and ideas are constantly changing, the clinical execution strength and time are also changing, while the curative effect is also changing. The above-mentioned suspicion, fear, laziness, and other negative emotions are the real causes of your illnesses. Therefore, the people who really heal themselves with PL are not only those who heal from diseases, but also those who improve their knowledge and habits. If your disease has improved but the knowledge and habits remain, you will often relapse. Usually there will be a relapse or the generation of a new illness.

The so-called self-healing shows that the self-healing force comes from oneself. Although it appears in the body, its source comes from the invisible mind. Although the natural medicine in the body is Qi, the source of life energy, it is controlled by the mind. In other words, the mind is the absolute head of the whole self-healing process. You can use a variety of tools to assist self-healing, strengthen the control of the mind to self-healing, but you must not fantasize with any external tools to replace the power of the mind. If you can enhance your confidence by Lajin bench, Paida stick, ginger jujube tea, red bean bag or functional bed sheet, heat source, etc., then there will be a positive effect. If the use of them makes you reduce PL times and become more dependent on the tools, then the tools have a negative effect. Because they weaken your enthusiasm, intensity, and time, and they lessen your inner true self-healing force. Drug users all know that drugs are harmful, but why do they want to take more and become addicted to them? It is precisely because drugs must have some effect to meet people's needs. It is this small benefit that makes people addicted and cannot extricate themselves. The long-term use will result in the loss of one's own natural function and more difficulty in activating the self-healing force. Then you will become increasingly dependent on external tools, drugs or characters, forming a vicious circle involuntarily.

The appearance of PL breaks the vicious cycle of human dependence on external forces for healing. These external forces have existed in the nice forms of helping people for thousands of years. They dazzle people. With excessive use, people will often be trapped by external forces, forgetting that their own internal strengths are already sufficient. The self-healing force from human self-reliance is both energy and information, which is far beyond the existing human insights, knowledge, and imagination. External power is only the product of finite human wisdom. It includes drugs, food, tools, experts etc. Certainly, I do not deny the role of these external forces, but I wish to remind mankind that the purpose and function of these external forces are also to pave the way for self-healing and remove obstacles. If you use them well, they will play a positive role, otherwise they will play a negative role.

So, long as we are still alive, our minds must direct the body to do clinical experiments. Everyone's way of life is the way of clinical experiments, and the experimental results will show up on the body. Therefore, the body has become the experimental tool and monitor of the mind. Physical illness is obviously the result of the wrong decision of the mind and has nothing to do with the body. Because the body cannot think, and it cannot make any decisions. In other words, being sick may be caused by choosing the wrong clinical approach, especially the way you see the world and yourself, namely your ideas and thoughts. As for certain, you can continue the previous clinical approach, which is actually your lifestyle, but if the disease is not healed after a long time, you can also add the Pl method to the lifestyle options. The purpose is to enhance your self-healing force, or it can be said to make the self-healing force that you have been suppressed in other ways to naturally present, to make you healthier and happier.

People accustomed to the old clinical way have long changed it into their own way of life, so they cannot help but doubt and fear a strange way. If the degree of simplicity and the effect of healing are far beyond their imagination, their doubt will be fiercer. Among the various doubts, the most significant one is that it has not been clinically verified, even if there are some successful cases, it is impossible to have a universal self-healing effect. The truth, however, is that clinical trials of PL have been done for 12 years, with thousands of experimenters around the world. The *Clinical Report of Paida and Lajin* is the statistics and summary of thousands of clinical experimental results we have collected.

Clinical experiments on healing should have been undertaken by doctors and scientists originally, but we have shouted and called for more than a decade, but they are still unwilling to do it. Thus, thousands of patients could not wait, they conducted themselves, and succeeded. It is reasonable to say that they were forced to become doctors and scientists. They published the results of their own experiments in a variety of ways, which can be regarded as constant emerging miracles. Facing such a vast number of positive results for more than a decade, however, no doctor, scientist or research institution has shown a little interest or curiosity. Isn't the spirit of science just exploration and discovery? Though I am not a scientist, I have more than a little bit of the spirit of scientific exploration and curiosity. Otherwise, the clinical reports written taking Pl friends' great energy and time cannot be arranged for research, and this scientific research that can save countless will continue to be buried in the human civilization formation of ignorance, darkness, and cruelty.

On what is a "scientific experiment", you can refer to an American monk's statement and get inspired. Before becoming a monk, he was a computer engineer in Silicon Valley.

The monk had suffered from back pain for years and remained in the hospital with no curing effect for a long time before becoming a monk. In the temple, he also tried acupuncture, massage, yoga, American chiropractic, and other external natural therapies for years, but gained little effect. Asking the cause, I just knew that it was from multiple sports injuries. He used to be a computer engineer working in Silicon Valley. He had developed a great interest in surfing and skiing since he was a student. However, he was injured many times and did not improve. With accumulations to now, the pain pierced through the whole back. He felt hurt even when sitting, and more painful when bending down or squatting. So, I asked two people to slap his back and the other the popliteal socket. He felt very painful when slapping, but he gritted his teeth and insisted. First, the palms were used to slap. After preheating, the Paida stick was applied, but he felt more pain! About 20 minutes with Paida and he was asked to get up and do all kinds of bending, squatting movements. He said happily that the pain had reduced to a half. Then I did a brief interview with him using a mobile phone video, which can still be watched on YouTube. He said this Paida alone was far better than dozens of previous treatments.

I was in this interview that he reminded me that the PL I did was a typical scientific experiment, and the results of this experiment should be published to benefit more people. I said a lot of people thought that only scientists can do scientific experiments. He replied, "What you have done is what scientists do, and the so-called scientific experiment is to record the results of the experiment. If the repeated experiment results are the same, you can prove that the method used is the scientific result. From what I have experienced and seen from the results; I dare to say that you are a genuine scientist." In fact, the motivation why I am now writing the *Clinical Report* has something to do with his encouragement at the time. Here I would like to thank him!

In order to eliminate the reading disorder formed by the old knowledge and reduce the strong impact of the *Pain Report* on people, I have to slightly hint and warm up the background and characteristics of this report. Although this report is a clinical summary of healing, it does differ from the paper you read in a medical journal. Its main features are as follows:

**I Clinical experimenters include both ordinary people and industry experts.**

In general, medical clinical experimenters are doctors and scientists. The people who do clinical experiments with PL are not medical experts. They come from all levels of society, and their medical knowledge is extremely limited. To be precise, they are patients. It is because their diseases that haven't been healed by doctors for so long that forces them to try this new clinical method.

Why are they called industry experts? Because they are practitioners of PL, they can become PL experts in repeated practice. The so-called clinical is relative to theoretical research. Although they are not theoretical experts, they are worthy experts in the field of clinical experiments. On the contrary, people who have not practiced PL do not have as much say in the clinical experiments of PL even if they have their own theoretical expertise.

**II The clinical experiment goal is not targeted at the specific disease, but the whole person.**

General medical clinical experiments deal with specific diseases. First, determine a certain drug and method that may heal a certain disease. Then list the relevant conditions and screen the qualified patients as experimental objects according to the standard. This method classifies the disease into a mode to facilitate instrumental measurement and physician analysis and diagnosis. So, simplified patterns replace complex symptoms, and they replace reality. Because people do not get sick according to the pattern, the real condition must be far more complicated than a simplified model. A disease name is an artificially defined label that depends on measurable, perceived limited indicators and is therefore misleading. With the progress of science and technology, medical instruments are more and more accurate in the detection of the human body, but it may be further away from the overall truth. Since the goal of this experiment is disease, not human, it often meets the indicators of treatment, but fails to make people healthy.

To get rid of this dilemma of clinical experiments, we must break through the practice of screening experimental subjects according to the name of the disease, not to treat a certain disease, but to target humans and set the overall physical and mental health as the standard. But not classified by name means that almost all human diseases can be healed. This idea alone has challenged existing human knowledge and beliefs, let alone doing experiments with it. However, the result of 12 years of millions of people doing the experiments is exactly like this: PL heals the whole person, not a certain disease. This formal change in clinical trials has included a breakthrough in medical theory. Obviously, doing experiments and observing human objects is more in line with the real situation, because everyone's state is unique. It is normal for a person to suffer from multiple diseases, and the diseases cannot be separated.

## III The randomness of clinical subjects raises the value of its medical statistics.

Since the goal of the experiment is the whole person rather than a certain disease, it means that anyone, no matter suffering how many diseases, can do clinical experiments with Pl. In other words, the experiment is full of randomness. Anyone, regardless of gender, age or disease, can apply PL. Initially it is only used for self-healing Paida, but soon it works on high blood pressure and heart disease. As the experimental number, the disease that PL can heal also increases. Even Alzheimer's disease, rheumatoid arthritis, cancer, diabetes, and other diseases have also been added to the healing list. Finally, the disease calculated from the clinical share statistics have reached hundreds, covering all the medical subjects.

The significant difference from the prior identification of the experiment is that the self-healing effective names are mostly known after the experiment. In other words, people constantly sent their own clinical reports to prove that a disease has recovered, no one thought in advance what PL can heal. It was just because someone happened to have the disease when doing the experiment and healed the disease with PL. This is random. For example, suffering regenerative anemia, people do not have blood creation function, and can only go regularly to the hospital for blood transfusion. This disease randomly appeared two times. One had blood transfusion for more than ten years, and one for two years. Both people recovered after PL, and the hematopoietic function was restored. Since the two cases appeared randomly, and only these two people of the same disease used the method, in terms of known cases, the medical statistical efficiency of such diseases is only 100%. Although the number of cases is not large, it is of great clinical value.

Another example comes to thyroid disease. There are dozens of cases of hyperthyroidism, hypothyroidism and thyroid tumor. PL was effective in all these cases. That is to say, the function of the thyroid was restored after PL, and the patients no longer take medicine. Two were diagnosed with thyroid cancer. They were operated on, a complete resection and partial resection respectively. Both cancer patients recovered their function after PL. The effect could not be reached by taking Levothyroxine Sodium Tablets. The partially removed thyroid gland actually regenerated and was healthy. There are only two cases of such cancer, but the success rate is 100%. This is not a preselection but is the result of a randomized clinic.

For example, gynecological disease cases involved 38 kinds of disease names, and a total of 613 cases. But it is 100% efficient for each disease, including more than 100 cases of irregular menstruation and breast hyperplasia. Therefore, I wonder if this makes people feel too exaggerated. It seems as if we have intended to raise it to such a high efficiency. But with more careful thinking, I think we should respect the facts, because these are all random cases. Moreover, even the nineteen breast cancers are 100% effective, some of which are cases of surgery and chemotherapy, which are the most difficult to treat, but the clinical results with PL are surprisingly wonderful. However, you can still see that the effect of PL is better for cancers without surgery and chemotherapy. But which case will appear more is unpredictable. They are all random.

Our clinical cases come from workshops, online workshops, groups of promoters of PL and individuals who practice Pl alone at home or with others. None of these cases come from hospital institutions and none are specially targeted at a certain disease. They are all targeted at humans and all cases randomly appear. As a result, they have high clinical values.

## IV The integrity and randomness of the PL targets make the disease names and divisions meaningless.

All clinical reports share a common feature, that is, while using PL for the purpose of healing a certain disease, the result turns out to be a surprise in that it healed several diseases actually or even more than ten maladies. Meanwhile, these diseases may belong to different departments. For instance, one set out to heal scapulohumeral periarthritis, but not only the scapulohumeral periarthritis healed, but high blood pressure also incidentally healed. For another example, one was ready to reduce blood pressure with PL, but found that diabetes mellitus, heart disease, and hyperthyroidism improved comprehensively. Or to treat leg pain and headache with PL, the result turned out to be that not only the leg pain and headache was resolved, even rhinitis, gastritis, and insomnia had been improved. It is especially true for patients suffering from all kinds of cancers. In addition to resolving cancer, overall improvements in more than ten other symptoms are common. For many patients who only have symptoms but cannot be diagnosed, PL has a unique advantage for it can often resolve the disease while both doctors and patients do not know the name. These cases are especially common in neurodegenerative conditions.

However, when I am preparing the Clinical Report, I classify generally according to the recognized diseases for the convenience of inquiry and discussion. But such classification, instead of a result of the clinical practice according to a preset mode, is the result of the random and extensive clinical practice. In other words, PL can be used to perform clinical experiments no matter who you are, what disease you are suffering or how many diseases are annoying you. Meanwhile, the diseases are healed for every one of many kinds, and I only classify cases with the same disease name or symptoms for discussion and study. But even though the disease name and malady are the same, the patient still suffers from other diseases and maladies. For this reason, the same case might appear in different classification reports. Such random experiments and classification are closer to the actual state. In the report with classification according to the disease name, I have tried my best to put a variety of cases with similar complications together to compare and discuss. For instance, diabetes patients are likely to have heart disease and high blood pressure, as well as leg disease, insomnia, frequent urination, gastrointestinal and other symptoms, or dysmenorrhea patients may have uterus, ovary, and breast disease, but they are all resolved or improved at the same time with PL.

If you have acquired the meaning of the integrity, randomness, and "forgetting the disease name" of clinical PL, you will find out that neglecting the medical division and disease name restrictions is just the key to self-healing with Pl. Because the disease that you want to heal does not exist alone. In fact, it interacts as both cause and effect with other diseases. Therefore, the specific disease that you want to heal can only be healed by improving all the other maladies. In, other words, the meaning of "forgetting the disease name" is only to let you forget the name of the disease rather than the disease itself. Meanwhile, the disease must be correlated with other diseases. As a result, forgetting the disease name reminds you that more known or unknown diseases will be improved with the disease. They rarely stand or fall alone. Obviously, this cannot be achieved through drugs because every drug has its target and function. Nonetheless, the reason that PL can resolve different diseases of different departments is that what it resolves is the common cause for all the maladies, that is, the blocked meridians.

This is beyond the understandable range of modern medicine, which has no concepts like meridians and Qi. Therefore, clinical experiment plays the role of verifying the above theory here, without clarifying into departments and regardless of disease names, can the method of PL be used to heal all the diseases? Do meridians and Qi really exist? The clinical discussion on the more than two hundred maladies involved in the clinical report with more than ten general classifications is to answer these questions exactly. We cannot void it only because doctors and scientists do not understand these phenomena and challenges. So, many maladies, like cancer, dementia, hypertension, and diabetes mellitus, which are hard to be through medical science can be healed without drugs. Isn't it the goal of medical science?

Whether a cold, stomach ache, cancer or depression, the applied clinical method is only to use the two simple movements of PL. It can be said that it proves the rule of "The greatest truths are the simplest". Whether people suffering from incurable terminal diseases, those annoyed by more than twenty kinds of diseases, infants, patients with depression that want to kill themselves or paraplegic patients who have to stayed in bed, in a word, people with complicated composite diseases in others' eyes and who have to take different medicines to deal with different maladies can use PL the clinical practice. Furthermore, regardless of the disease name, or the different degrees of difficulty in people's views, PL makes no exception. It uses the two simple movements to cope with everything.

This kind of minimalist clinical practice is actually the verification of the theory of minimalist PL, that is, all diseases are from the blocked meridians, so getting through the meridians is self-healing. Seriously ill and weak people always think of nutrition, and PL theory also tells that getting through meridians means great nutrition. It is this minimalist theory and minimalist clinical experiments that can simplify extremely complex minds and diseases. This simplification cannot be learned by theory alone but must only be achieved in clinical experiments.

**V The clinical practice of PL has holographic and integrated features.**

The reason why the PL experiment can ignore the name, the seriousness of diseases and the number of diseases is that the self-healing force activated by it has holographic and integrated features. Because self-healing force is a kind of energy beyond human imagination, or Qi, and each unit contains holographic and holistic information. Therefore, its healing is not for a local or certain symptom but aims at the overall health of the whole person. However, the invisible characteristic of self-healing force is quite mysterious, as if it will be made from nothing with PL. And in fact, it is indeed out of nothing, because the eyes can only see tangible things, and real life is invisible. Self-healing is from nature. It belongs to the spiritual level, while people's knowledge cannot reach the holographic and integrated state, but its diagnosis and healing effect is obvious through HC. Thus, humans will gradually get used to this mysterious feature in clinical practice.

**VI The clinical reports of PL have unique styles, but consistent conclusion.**

Because these clinical reports are the sharing of ordinary people on the effect of PL. They are neither professional doctors nor scientists, and obviously they will not write reports according to the usual paper style. They have different styles. So, they focus on the clinical process, such as PL methods, HC, and emphasize their medical and healing history. But regardless of their styles, it does not affect the most valuable information of the clinical report, that is, superior efficacy. And efficacy is the most important concern for all patients.

In fact, it is precisely because the reports are written by ordinary patients, and they are both the clinical implementers and the objects of implementation, that is, the implementer and the object are one, that their feelings about PL are more profound and sincere, they feel profounder about the advantages and disadvantages of PL and the reports are more real and touching. Many people were moved after reading the PL reports of senior PL friends, and just took the road of PL, and soon output their own reports. It is exactly because they are not medical experts but ordinary patients that their words and feelings are closer to every reader, giving them empathy and inspiring the self-healing force that everyone has.

In brief, these reports are the sincere and frank sharing of every patient from the bottom of theirs hearts, thus endowing them with power. In fact, the mind is the only thing that can be really shared in the world. It will not be on the decrease like tangible things while sharing, but more and more, and with greater resonance, sympathy and resultant force. Because the seemingly separated countless different minds derive from the same source and are actually the same one, which is where the truth of the soul lies.

In addition to the conclusion of self-healing disease that is obvious to people and another conclusion that almost all PL friends come to, is that the clinical practice of PL has changed their knowledge and emotions, that is, improved their spiritual diseases. Since PL should be determined by the heart from beginning to end, and the spiritual disease has been producing a variety of HC, the improvement of the spiritual disease is naturally without suspense. Because PL are self-healing, the patient's own mind then restores the role of a real doctor unknowingly. The patient has an unprecedented new perception of the cause and healing in the clinic and understands the true meaning of the disease from the heart and curing the disease by the heart. Thus, PL, the convenient method of self-healing also paves the way for cultivating the spirit. Therefore, whether you believe in Buddhism, Taoism, Jesus, yoga, Qigong and other kinds and explore on the spiritual road, you will find that PL has become your aid and convenient method for your spiritual cultivation.

Conclusion: I intended to classify and statistics for the PL cases and data collected according to the names of the diseases, and then analyze and discuss them originally, so as to achieve an obvious self-healing law. However, with the deepening research on various disease cases and the comparative discussion with monographs written by western medicine experts, it is found that general statistics and principal discussion are far from enough to satisfy readers' curious desire for the details of the clinical process.

Therefore, I made up my mind to classify all cases according to the disease names. In addition to classifying clinical efficacy statistics, each clinical case was analyzed one by one and discussed and compared with similar cases to meet the various needs of curious people and critics.

Taking "stroke" as an example, the cases will be comprehensively listed one by one for discussion according to the order of precursor of stroke, ictal stroke, stroke and has been admitted to hospital, stroke and has used surgery or drug treatment, and stroke sequelae.

For "diabetes", the completely stopped insulin, completely stopped drugs, halved medication and other cases are listed so that people can see that drug dependence of a variety of different degrees can be completely stopped successfully while the rehabilitation is achieved.

For "gynecological disease", the irregular menstruation and menopause syndrome, dysmenorrhea, uterine lesions, infertility and pregnancy disease, ovarian disease, postpartum disease, and breast disease are classified as listed into a total of seven chapters, with each chapter showing many vivid and wonderful cases.

For "hypertension", the common hypertension, complex hypertension, high-risk hypertension, and extremely high-risk hypertension are arranged in turn for case discussion, because of its gradually increasing complications until the extremely high-risk degree.

Some diseases are discussed in western medicine monographs, such as pain and depression, so they are discussed with other similar PL cases. Thus, *Pain and Depression: A Comparison of Western Medicine and PL Clinical Cases* is output.

Currently, the finished related reports include:

"Clinical report of PL applied in hypertension / hypotension", "Stroke clinical report", "Nephropathy clinical report", "Diabetes clinical report", "Lung and respiratory disease clinical report", "Lung and gastrointestinal disease clinical report", "Lung and skin disease clinical report", "Gynecological disease clinical report",

"Depression and mood disease clinical report", "Pain and depression: A comparison of western medicine and PL clinical cases", "Thyroid disease clinical report", "Cancer and tumor clinical report", "Hepatobiliary disease clinical report", "Neurodegenerative disease clinical report", as well as "Deafness and tinnitus clinical report". Clinical reports of other conditions will follow as the cases increase.

Clinical reports not prepared according to the standards of medical papers seem not to meet the scientific standards, which is a disadvantage. But from another point of view, it is a great advantage, because each case is a true story, and some stories are more wonderful than movies and novels. Hence, it does not matter if you don't regard them as clinical reports, at least they can bring you some entertainment, which will help you to clear the meridians and improve your mood. You can even disbelieve any of the principles and efficacy of PL, but you should at least trust the sincere record and sharing of each author and feel their compassion and kindness. They are not doctors and the reason they try to write these words about healing is only to help you and your family to get rid of pain and embrace happiness earlier. Clinical experiments are not about theory, but about exploring the results of discovery with action, experience, and facts. Their writing may be very unprofessional, but their simplicity and kindness are touching.

For example, a stroke patient was unconscious and unable to breathe his last breath due to discomfort. The nurse looked at the patient and waited silently for the final outcome so as to decide whether to push the patient back to the ward or to the morgue. At this time, the author finally felt unbearable, regardless of the taboo of the hospital, when the two nurses were present, practiced Paida on the elbow socket of the father, that is, the dying patient with great strength! Only with this action, Sha appeared in chaos, and the patient exhaled a long breath on the spot. He was saved from significant risk...

Another example is that a woman's mother suffered diabetes, heart disease and other diseases that broke out at the same time and ended up in hospital with various pipelines inserted on the whole body. She was weak. The lady rushed to the ward, regardless of the doctor's opposition, and practiced Paida on her mother. Sha appeared on the whole body, and she could get up on the spot and independently walk more than ten layers downstairs. So, other patients and their families filled the room and lined up for her to practice PL...

There was a lady whose mammary gland tumor had been large enough to occupy two-thirds of the breast and was hard as a stone. Her mother-in-law, as a doctor, had her admitted to hospital for surgery, but she and her mother insisted on Paida. She not only patted the whole body and patted the tumor to a soft state with septic blood. Then the lesion automatically bursts out of pus and blood. She recovered in less than two months. But there were small lumps that were just checked out and the patients who were afraid then had surgery but suffered more sequelae...

There were also patients with femoral head necrosis, diabetes patients, or psoriasis, who, after a long treatment without effect, healed their chronic and stubborn diseases with PL and then become the disseminators of PL as well as professional Paida masters. One of the most legendary characters is Master Cao, a patient originally suffering from a variety of serious illnesses. Since all the symptoms healed with Pl, he has been teaching PL for people every evening in Beibei Park, ChongQing, voluntarily. There are more than tens of thousands of patients all over the country who come for learning. You will find many self-healing cases of incurable diseases in this report.

The above are just a few examples, for more clinical cases or wonderful stories, you need to explore, discover, appreciate and entertain in this *Clinical Report of Pain and Lajin*. As for certain, the most intoxicating and enjoyable way of entertainment is your own clinical trials with PL. Perhaps besides obtaining entertainment, you will be the next one to write a clinical report!

——Hongchi Xiao, on October 25, 2022

# Several terms concerning the Clinical Report of PL

As it is the first time for many people to hear about PL Self-healing, I will explain a few main terms related to this method to help you better understand the Clinical Report. The specific cases you are about to read are the most vivid interpretations of these terms. The clinical discussion of each case also continues to explore the meaning of these concepts from different perspectives. To find a more detailed theoretical interpretation of them, you can refer to the *Paida and Lajin Self-healing*.

## 1. What is Paida and Lajin?

Paida is to slap certain parts of the body or even the whole body in the strength you can endure with your hand or some tool. The time you spend on Paida can last from a few minutes to several hours, depending on your own decision. Meanwhile, you can also perform Paida with each other for better effect. Lajin refers to pulling the limbs and body in different postures. The most common posture reported is the recumbent position, that is, lying on your back, with one leg upright, leaning on a post or door frame, and the other leg naturally lowered; another posture is Y-shaped Lajin, that is, lying on the bed or the floor, leaning your legs against the wall, and trying your best to pull your legs to both sides, just like a Y-shape. Other postures include squatting, standing with hands raised, standing on a Lajin board and gradually raising the angle of your toes, and so on.

Both methods have been inherited for fitness and healing by the Chinese folk for thousands of years. They are simple and can be mastered in minutes. Their curative effects depend on the duration and intensity of implementation. In general, the longer the duration and the greater the intensity, the better the efficacy. Combining the two methods works better, so they are integrated and called PL. It is much simpler than the familiar Tai Chi, yoga and general sports. In reports, it is named PL for short.

## 2. What is Qi? What are meridians?

Qi is the life energy inherent in the human body, which is called "Qi" in Chinese, but can only be interpreted as an electromagnetic wave by modern science. Instead of merely life energy, Qi also contains life information beyond human recognition, so let's just call it holography. The self-healing or healing power we call is basically made up of Qi. It detaches from the body, belongs to none of the body parts, and is formless and faceless, so the understanding of it in modern science is limited. However, this does not impede mankind from making full use of it and continuing to explore and discover it. PL is a convenient way to heal yourself with Qi.

It can be known from the meridian theory of traditional Chinese medicine and the Indian yoga tradition that the smooth movement of Qi in the body will lead to the health of the human body, while if the movement of Qi is slowed down or even completely stagnated, various diseases will be generated in your body. Qi, rather than moving irregularly, runs in a given channel, which is called a "meridian" in Chinese medicine and "chakra" in yoga. Both PL and yoga are aimed at getting through the channels of Qi, namely meridians. However, Chinese medicine focuses on curing diseases, while yoga stresses spiritual enlightenment.

Traditional Chinese medicine and yoga pay more attention to the energy field in the human body composed of Qi, namely the energy body, rather than the chemical body, which Western medicine focuses on more.

## 3. What are the HC?

PL directly stimulate the human body to activate and strengthen the rate and quantity of flow of Qi in the body, exerting impact on various diseases developed in the body, and forming a variety of physical, chemical, and physiological reaction symptoms, namely HC ( QiChong BingZao in Chinese ). It means that the clogged meridians are being unblocked by Qi. The most common symptoms are pain and Sha that almost everyone will encounter. In addition, other reactions of HC include sweating, burping, farting, itching, eruption, vomiting, dizziness, fatigue, palpitation, broken skin with tissue fluid, bleeding, blisters, clumps, dark urine, abnormal stool and so on. And you can see that the common feature they share is the elimination of disease and virus in the body which are formed by energy impacts, so they can be called energy markers.

The seemingly unpleasant HC is first an accurate diagnosis. You can compare the symptoms of HC with the slapped meridians to determine which meridians are blocked, and what poisons exist in the body. Secondly, healing also occurs simultaneously with HC. Some people are frightened by the HC, mistaking the reward as a punishment. Because if there is no disease in the body, a HC will never appear. And the disease is exactly what Paida wants to find and resolve. Observing HC is the key to discussing clinical cases of pain.

For further understanding, please read Steve's; "The Healing Wisdom of PL ——HC (Reactions)".

**The Healing Wisdom of PL——HC**

HC (simplified as HC) is the human body's reaction that occurs during and after doing PL (slapping and stretching or simplified as PL) and that is why it's also called HC. It is the key to understanding PL Self-Healing. In fact, it is the way or path to self-healing, but it is also a myth.

PL self-healing for me is about conditioning the body. So, our mind does not stand in the way of developing healing consciousness and HC HC is the awareness of PL self-healing with its ability to detox, heal and prevent diseases. HC becomes visible through exercising PL self-healing. Is this a weird statement to you? My first understanding of HC, I encountered by reading Hongchi Xiao's book *Paid and Lajin Self-Healing*. I thought I understood it then but not really. So, allow me to reconnect you with my personal experience and present understanding of HC.

Even though I find myself in prison and am limited in area and am confined in a cell for 19 hours a day and am restricted to 3-5 hours outside time in our prison yard. I still practice PL self-healing and we have no luxury of having a Lajin bench or something as simple as a hand slapper. The feeling of knowing no limitation can stop me by only using my hands and the prison table outside in the prison yard is gratifying enough. The confined space of my cell and the prison yard are my personal workshop areas for practicing PL self-healing.

It has been more than 14 months since I have been exercising PL self-healing with my bare essentials, my hands. My initial awareness of HC was for me more than a crisis; its experience presented more of a phenomenon, something unknown and invisible. Its healing consciousness was as if my body was searching and experiencing feelings after doing PL slapping and stretching. After reading Hongchi's book on self-healing, it gave me a clearer understanding of HC an insight to why I was experiencing symptoms of pain, swelling, severe itchiness and the visible evidence of "Sha". It gave me a personal understanding of HC and its powerful effect on my physical and emotional transformation.

These feelings and sensations became something I wanted to share with Hongchi on a daily basis for my personal insight and understanding. So, every day I ask Hongchi why I am experiencing such a heavy deep release of physical, emotional pressure. Our sharing became a feeling of gratitude and a personal understanding of this phenomenon which is HC.

There is nothing normal about prison, it is a cruel and desperate place but to have something such as PL self-healing and to be able to exercise and heal yourself is a relief and joy. The transformation that it creates in my physical well-being is a miracle. I can see and feel the transformation and become deeply conscious that I must go through something known and unknown – this is HC. This occurring transformation not only gave me strength that I had not experienced for a long time, but surprisingly also gave me confidence and joy.

HC HC uncovered in me a lot of hidden sickness and created feelings and sensations which are hard to describe and name. Like the first time I slapped my waist area, both front and back, the pain, swelling and "sha" that appeared was so strange. It looked just like "crocodile skin". Very dark, lumpy rough "sha" which is a very swollen and throbbing sensation. Over more than one week, I would watch the changes, the "sha" changed color three times from a deep purple to dark red than a mixture of blue, red and yellow. I would say to Hongchi my thoughts as if some crocodile ghost or demon is trying to escape out of my body prison, how ironic, hahaha. My slapping and stretching have created a lot of different HC symptoms, these are some of the symptoms I experienced:-

1. Pain and numbness
2. Sha
3. Bleeding
4. Itchiness
5. Swelling
6. Sweating
7. Vomiting
8. Fatigue
9. Smelly Body Odor
10. Bloody Nasal Mucus
11. Deep throbbing sensation

These are the initial and first symptoms that appear that made me realize that I have disease and sickness. These are the visible signs of HC. This is how my body responded to PL self-healing which I believe gives me the experience and understanding our diseases and sickness are deep rooted. These signs are physical evidence. The experience HC is the different feelings and sensations. My analogy of this is something like a feeling of "Hidden ghosts inside".

Prison has given me the opportunity to reconnect with myself, by practicing PL self-healing with Hongchi most days. It has become a daily ritual and a part of prison life.

My awareness tells me HC is the only mechanism that activates the receptors of the brain, and the body reveals the true effects of self-diagnosis. I do not know the body's wisdom of how it heals and balances itself, but I know I am experiencing a feeling of recovery and witnessing a holistic transformation because I no longer use the medications that I have been using for several years prior to my imprisonment and starting my journey with PL self-healing.

I have come to realize after all these years of using medications that it only relieves pain and suffering and does not really heal the root cause of any of my diseases and sickness but only maintains their cause by suppressing the deep roots of my diseases as hidden ghosts in my body.

Slapping always reveals visible HC known as "Sha". This is deep rooted; manifested disease I find in me that appears in different forms, shapes and textures. For me, it is a natural sign that my body is self-diagnosing, detoxing, healing, and preventing many different unknown diseases.

Pain, sha, swelling and itchiness are always present, with every session of slapping no matter what part of my body. My understanding is the longer the duration and intensity of my slapping, the more HC initiates healing and activates the prevention of whatever the unknown disease and this prevention is imminent. Why? Because when one of the HC symptoms no longer appears, this means that HC has reached its peak. Which means the symptoms are declining and diminishing with a healing effect at the same time.

For me, this is how HC gives me the sign that I am improving in my health and having more energy and greater endurance of pain. My slapping has become a lot stronger and more intense, and I can stretch past 90 degrees in my Lajin stretching.

My awareness has become that PL self-healing generates and transforms energy. It is this feeling of different sensations that vibrates through me when I slap and give me a feeling unknown, as if the sickness is being shaken and chased out of my body. This vibration that is created by PL is the heart of HC. This shows why HC is the "way" of recovery and the key to understanding PL self-healing.

HC HC reveals different hidden diseases and illnesses that are known and many unknowns that linger in our bodies as past afflictions.

HC HC is the "BULLSHIT DETECTOR" of my suffering and this affliction PL is something so simple and this is why the world cannot easily fathom its healing effect. That's why it can only be understood by those who have experienced its healing effects. Sadly, even the world media has portrayed PL self-healing in an opaque screen of concepts, labels, images, words, judgments and definitions. The media's portrayal in my view is ignorant and biased, it is lacking in research, experience and understanding but I know the truth will prevail. This is not only the will of myself and Hongchi, but also the will of all the PL families and that of the greater will above us all.

PL self-healing in its simplicity and wordless understanding can only be administered by our own actions, the actions of slapping and stretching. To this present day and a time of more than 14 months practicing PL in prison, all of us in our prison workshop still experience significant HC indicators of pain, sha, swelling and itchiness, for me this detox mainly is more sensitive on my hands and feet. One of my very first experiences was bleeding on my hands, stained by a thick white powder, severe swelling and heavy "sha", this also happened to my feet. As HC started to diminish the varicose veins on my hands and feet were gone. Another healing was my mouth cancer, this was most unexpected. In prison help is hard to come by and is very limited, almost non-existent for a disease such as mouth cancer. So, Hongchi advised me to try (Paida) slapping. I started with very light slapping; the pain was severe, intolerable and went all the way into my heart. I continued to slap my mouth and whole head at intervals of 10-15 minutes. My lips started to sting and swell. My lower lip cracked open and started to bleed in 2 different places, my lips turned deep purple. The strongest sensation was a deep throbbing and pinching pain, it would wake me in my sleep. The feeling was as if someone was trying to dig the cancer out with a sharp knife. I could feel my cancer all over the inside of my mouth with my tongue. It felt like hard strings or tendons on the inside of my cheeks and lower lip. This is the awareness of HC. Even though most of the sensations and tangible signs have diminished, my mouth no longer cracks and bleeds after slapping. I still feel slight throbbing after slapping but the pinching pain at night is gone. I can confidently say my mouth cancer has improved by 80 percent. The best thing is I do not have to have an operation to cut the cancer from my mouth.

Vomiting is a significant symptom of HC. It happened to me on three different occasions, the most obvious was after slapping my mouth and both sides of my neck and my belief is due to my mouth cancer because it happened so unexpectedly. My mouth and throat would always be dry and no matter how much water or tea I would drink it could not quench my thirst. Since vomiting on three occasions, yellow sticky mucus, I felt an instant relief in my throat and chest. The next morning, I blew a thick brown paste from my nose filled with thick blood. After a few minutes my nose started to ooze out clear liquid for several hours and stopped. I think all these HC symptoms are deep rooted and related to my cancer and other unknown diseases but now the feeling of dry mouth and throat are gone, and I no longer wheeze when I breathe or snore in my sleep. This is how HC diminishes and prevents diseases. This is a detox of deep-rooted sicknesses and diseases.

Exercising PL self-healing and experiencing HC is like an awakening for me. To explain it to you is so notoriously hard in words which brings me to a realization that really all healing experiences like this type of phenomenon are hard to describe. It can only be explained if the person I am talking with is familiar with the same experience. So, I must rely on your experience of PL self-healing is similar for you as it is for me. Only then can the truth be shared between us.

This prison journey has been rather exceptional; I have Hongchi who has shared his wisdom and existentialism of PL self-healing with me. His wisdom has given me a conditioning of the mind which brings me to the importance of meditation as a key component of PL self-healing.

Meditation is the path to healing the heart. Meditation is the actionless and thoughtless process of PL self-healing and HC is the awareness and understanding of inner change physically, emotionally and spiritually. Meditation gives me inner strength and conditioning when I am slapping myself or somebody else. Meditation gives me a deeper understanding of HC.

HC is not all pain and suffering, it also consists of joy, gratitude, forgiveness and feeling of compassion but for me it consists mainly of awareness of self, my authentic self. It is the feeling of joy watching myself change inside and outside. HC HC activates the body's healing wisdom by us experiencing, verifying, and proving the results of our healing. This is the truth of HC for me; it is like walking the path of the healing heart. What I have noticed in myself is the more I exercise PL self-healing, the more HC diminishes and the more my energy level increases, I am able to withstand longer periods of slapping and my tolerance to pain has greatly increased. Furthermore, my eyesight has improved, I no longer wear my prescription glasses regularly and I have minimal heart pain. These are only some of the joys of my recovery of better health practicing PL self-healing.

The biggest gratitude I give to PL self-healing is for stopping the use of all my prescribed medications and supplements. I am prescribed medication for high blood pressure, elevated sugar glucose levels, arthritis pain and inflammation. I took supplements for my joints, mainly my knees and ankles and used creams for swelling. I use creams for my eczema. My skin used to be very dry and flaky like dandruff, with red rashes on my arms and legs which were painful and itchy for days. No one asked me to stop medications, but I made the decision myself after I started doing PL self-healing.

As PL self-healing and HC go hand in hand all these mentioned symptoms and sensations are all gone, my blood pressure and glucose level are normalized, and my skin condition has disappeared as if by some sort of miracle. For me this is detox, healing and preventing diseases and the power of PL self-healing and how I recognize HC.

Sometimes I wonder what the difference between disease is and HC. I have come to the realization it is the same thing but appears in different ways. My analogy of disease is, it is like a hidden bomb waiting to explode and then it explodes the damage is irreparable. If it is a small explosion the damage is small. It could be something like a stroke, heart attack or some sort of cancer. we can survive for a better period but if a bigger bomb explodes like a nuclear bomb. There is no recovery, damage that is if you are dead. As we say in prison "You are fucked". My analogy is direct or even a little bit crude, but it is true. The effects of HC have made me aware as a sick person. I surely have more HC than a healthier person which also reveals if I have no HC there would be no disease or sickness, and all HC is always related to some sort of blockage in the body.

This is my blessing and gift from the Holy One to be able to share these last 14 months with Hongchi Xiao exercising PL self-healing. PL PL is not only healing me physically. It has given me a greater understanding of mental, emotional and spiritual awareness. I now know that all my diseases and illnesses are derived from self-inflicted mental and emotional stress and false beliefs. Fear, Anger, Depression, Worries, self-neglect are only a few I dare to name. So, my heart became my focus, all my heart felt negative emotions are the cause of all my physical and mental diseases.

PL self-healing has transformed me emotionally with a feeling of unconditional
Love for myself.   HC is a personal inner change. A wonderful feeling in the heart that follows me as a constant companion of calm and humility. It is about shrinking the suffering thoughts, emotions, anxieties, and fears which upset my sense of harmony that prevents my healthier state of self-improvement.

As a person changing my relationship with myself in this world is the key which also helps to sidestep the everyday dangers of prison life. I am suffering due to life pressures in my incarceration; this imprisonment is keeping me away from my family.

In finding Hongchi and exercising PL self-healing through the effects and awareness of HC my physical and mental toxins are being cleansed in a natural and non-medicated way. I will continue my self-healing after my release from prison and look forward to more favorable circumstances but for now I will continue with my deeper understanding of PL self-healing and the significance of HC.

HC is about protecting the body. You must become aware PL provides healing. PL PL healing is from the "heart". Awareness of understanding what we have to understand and experiencing what we have to experience.

The path of the healing heart is love and love always provides healing, and the feeling of love is the presence of the "Holy One" or "Dao".

Be grateful whenever the presence of the Holy One is demonstrated through self-healing and the power of PL. Stay with the heart, the "life energy" of Dao.

To heal this world, this planet—every individual's journey is an integral part of the life journey of all beings. The journey of our planet and the whole universe, each person has the sacred responsibility to engage in healing themselves and healing the world.

This points to a deeper understanding why healing ourselves, healing the world means healing our relationship with the world. It is our relationship that needs to be repaired; our relationship with our physical, emotional, and spiritual self and experience tells us that healing relationships call for inner change. Now this inner change is the sacred responsibility that becomes apparent which is the healing of our individual self. In other words, the healing of our relationship with our body and authentic self.

Healing, the world depends upon healing and transformation of each person. Through PL self-healing as you become aware of your physical self, you will realize that each person is sacred and the planet and the whole world. Our awareness becomes that we are healing our relationship with these aspects of creation. Though we are the embodiment of the Creator we may find it hard to accept that we have everything we need within us for self-healing. Our bodies are all aspects of the Holy One/Dao and the Holy One expresses life through us.

A flower is the Holy One being a flower. An ant is the Holy One being an ant. A human being is the Holy One being a human being. Awareness is so hard to put into words.

Walking the path of the heart with PL self-healing. It takes discipline, strength and courage to accept PL self-healing. It is accepting the truth of who we are and knowing the presence of the Holy One. We find it easier to avoid looking closely at ourselves because we have unconsciously accepted the images and stereotypes created by our families, society, religion and culture.

A self-healer is someone who walks the path of the heart. Understanding, experiencing and accepting his or her true nature. Knowing the dark and light live together in the heart!

The path of the heart takes us deep into awareness of self-healing, deep into life, our own life, the life of others, the life of the earth and finding the love of the Holy One living inside. Healing our soul is the bridge over the chasm and finding our authentic self. This is the hidden secret in all of us. So, let me conclude with something I would like you to contemplate a riddle for all of you PL practitioners, followers and foes of PL self-healing. What cannot be seen? What cannot be heard? What cannot be touched? What cannot be thought?

Pain and suffering will appear and diminish as HC in your meditation and awareness.

What is it that cannot be seen but which makes seeing possible?

What is it that cannot be heard but which makes hearing possible?

What is it that cannot be known but which makes knowledge possible?

What is it that cannot be thought but which makes thinking possible?

As an existentialist HC is a deep awakening, a deep knowing of our deep authentic self. This is awareness, a consciousness you cannot see, hear or touch, and it is extremely mysterious. You can experience it, feel it, you know it is in you – this is awareness.

Only awareness experiences seeing but has no color or shape.
Only awareness experiences hearing but makes no sound.
Only awareness experiences touching but has no tangible form.
Only awareness experiences thinking but is not a thought.

HC is awareness of how PL self-healing transforms us physically, mentally, emotionally, and spiritually. This is Hongchi Xiao's PL self-healing and my experience and understanding.

——Srebre Ordan Todoroski    27/12/2018

## 4. What is Sha?

Sha refers to the toxins and wastes discharged by the human body due to HC. The most common forms of HC are pain and Sha. During PL, the more in pain you are, and the more Sha appears, it means the more the meridians are blocked. It is easy to understand what pain is because everyone has different feelings about it. However, it is not the case for Sha. Superficially, Sha is the various colors presented on the skin after Paida. In general, it appears as red, and then gradually turns dark red, purple and black gradually, in the shape of a small particle, piece, lump etc. Therefore, people generally mix it up with the bruises caused by injury. In fact, they differ from each other essentially.

Sha, instead of the bruise caused by trauma impact, is a pathological substance formed by the chemical reaction between the stimulated Qi and the pathogen and virus in the body. It is more easily dissolved and expelled from the body. So, you can see that the elimination of toxicants by HC will not move the toxicant from one place to another just like cleaning the rubbish. It will impact the pathogen with Qi and react with it in a chemical way to turn the pathogen into a new substance that can be decomposed more easily. Then, the pathogen can be expelled from appropriate outlets, such as sweat pores, excrement and emiction.

Other natural therapies known to people, such as Cupping and Skin scraping also produce Sha. They share the same nature. However, Paida can produce various kinds of Sha with deep colors, which makes it incomparable to other therapies. In like manner, other therapies cannot match Paida in the produced types and intensity of HC. This is one of the reasons that Paida has powerful self-healing.

## 5. What are the main meridians in the human body? Where are they distributed in the body?

There are twelve main meridians in our human body, which are called the twelve regular meridians. They are distributed in the four limbs, connected to the viscera in the body and named after the relevant viscera. Among them, six are located on the hands and arms, three for Yin and three for Yang. The other six are on the feet and legs, also three for Yin and three for Yang. They are all symmetric. Meanwhile, there are two meridians in the median lines of human chests and backs. They are named Ren-meridian and Du-meridian. As a result, some people add the two meridians up and consider them as 14 meridians in the human body.

Those lie on the palms and the inner sides of arms are heart meridian, pericardium meridian, and lung meridian. The heart meridian connects with the little finger, the lung meridian associates with the thumb and the pericardium meridian is in the middle. The three meridians are three Yin meridians. They get through the heart, lung and pericardium in the chest. At the back of the hands and the outside of the arm exist the large intestine meridian, small intestine meridian and Sanjiao meridian. The three meridians are three Yang meridians. They run along the outer sides of arms, and part into two branches in the shoulder and neck part. One enters the abdomen to connect with the large intestine and small intestine, while the other passes the neck to connect with the head and the five sense organs. As a result, you can heal from your diseases in the digestive system as well as on the head and face by slapping the back of the hands and the outer sides of arms.

On the inner sides of the legs, there are three Yin meridians, namely, the liver meridian, spleen meridian and kidney meridian, which connect to the three viscera respectively. On the outer sides of the legs, there are gallbladder and stomach meridians, while the bladder meridian exists on the back of the legs. The three are Yang meridians connected with the three organs respectively. On the instep, from the side of the great toe outwards, there are the liver meridian, stomach meridian and gallbladder meridian in parallel. Under the medial foot and medial malleolus, they are the meridians of kidney and spleen. On the inner sides of the feet and under the malleolus medialis, there are the renal meridian and spleen meridian. Besides, the bladder meridian is on the outer sides of the feet and under external malleolus. The three Yang meridians, namely the bladder meridian, gallbladder meridian, and stomach meridian, besides being connected with namesake organs, also associate with the head and face. The three Yang meridians of the hand and the foot are connected with the head and face, so slapping the hands and feet are not only to treat the disease in the viscera but also to treat those on the head and face.

For the convenience of memory, you can remember them in the abridged way as follows:

The heart, lung, and pericardium meridians are on the inner sides of the arms while the large intestine, small intestine and Sanjiao meridians are on the outer sides of the arms.

The liver, spleen, and kidney meridians are on the inner sides of the legs, the gallbladder and stomach meridians are on the outer sides of the legs while the urinary bladder meridian is at the back of the legs.

It won't be a big deal if you can't remember them, because you must slap the four limbs first to heal all the maladies yourself. And then you can slap the head and the body. Therefore, you only need to remember the four limbs. Meanwhile, the elbow section is always the start point of Paida. There are not a few people who have already healed their diseases without making clear meridians.

So, you can see that it is more important to slap the whole body than to remember meridians.

## 6. What are the Universal Parts?

If you cannot remember meridians, this method will be more convenient, effort-saving and timesaving for you. As the term suggests, universal means that Paida on these parts can be commonly applied for all maladies.

The universal parts include the elbows, the hands, the knees and the feet, showing that they are the major joint parts on the limbs. Obviously, to remember the four parts is much easier than to remember the traditional Chinese medicine acupoints. Actually, there are eight universal parts all together on the two sides of the human body as it has two hands and two feet. In fact, if you have slapped the universal parts, it means that you have reached all the twelve regular meridians. Meanwhile, most of the important acupoints exist on the universal parts. However, please note that you cannot slap merely one side of the universal parts. You need to slap each side like both the inner and outer sides of the elbow, the front, the back, the left and the right sides of the knee, the palm and the back sides of the hand, as well as the instep, the internal ankle, external ankle and the sole sides of the foot.

If you do not have much time, you can slap the universal parts and then gradually slap the four limbs and the whole body. Paida covers a wider range than acupuncture. After you slap once, in fact, you have worked on all the meridians. Let's see an example. If you have slapped the chelidon (inside of the elbow), it means that you have reached the heart, lung, and pericardium meridians at the same time.

# Introduction

The symptoms of thyroid disease are well understood by Western medicine. It can only be said that there is a problem with the immune system that leads to a disruption of thyroid secretion. Why is there a problem with the immune system? How can it be improved? If the cause is clarified by medical research, the problem would have been solved. Since the advent of PL method, the clinical trials with patients have demonstrated that the cause of thyroid disease is no different from any other disease, it is simply a blockage of the meridians. The main cause of the blockage of the meridians is the mind, which includes the negative emotions and mmisunderstandings.

For more information on the relationship between heart disease and thyroid disease, please refer to the introduction to the *Clinical Report of PL on Gynecological Disorders*. In short, thyroid disorders are manifestations of heart disorders in the body in the different places and ways, as gynecological disorders. Because of the strong association between two types of illnesses and negative emotions, gynecological illnesses and thyroid illnesses often occur together in one person. It is not difficult to observe another phenomenon, namely that people with these types of illness have various degrees of depression. It is only that some are diagnosed, and others are not yet known. They know whether they are happy in their minds or not. Men also also suffer from thyroid disease, but to a lesser degree. The causes are the same as for women.

Since thyroid problems are linked to the immune system, we must figure out the specific reason that the immune system is out of order. Why are some people strong and others weak? In short, the immune system is part of the self-healing system or self-healing power. The strength of the immune system depends on the smoothness of the meridians. The clearer the meridians and the more positive energy the body has, the stronger the immune system will be. You can read more cases and discussions related to inflammation and immune disorders in *Pain and Depression: A Comparative Western and PL Clinical Report*. These simple principles can also be verified by all clinical cases in this report.

Which kinds of meridian blockages cause this disease? There is no doubt that all illnesses are compound illnesses. Therefore, all 12 main meridians of the body are usually blocked, and it is logical that the PL of whole body should be used for self-healing. However, there is a pattern. Since the disease is triggered by heart disease, first depression will cause blockages in the heart, pericardium, and lung meridians; secondly, in the three Yang meridians of the hand, i.e. the small intestine, Tri-jiao and large intestine meridians on the outside of the arm. These six meridians (three Yang and three Yin meridians) of the hand also intersect with the thyroid gland. Besides, there are three Yin Meridians of the feet, which are related to blood, namely the liver, spleen and kkidney meridians, which are cognate to these three meridians: bladder, stomach and gallbladder meridians.

# Chapter 1 Statistical report of thyroid disease cases treated with PL

A total of 41 cases of thyroid disease PL with text sharing have been collected, of which 39 cases were women and 2 cases were men.

The sources of the cases are shown as below:

1. Clinical reports written by participants of PL workshops.
2. Clinical reports written by patients themselves after studying and experimenting with PL from books and the Internet.
3. Clinical reports written by group members of online PL groups around the world after the experiments of PL.

Although their reports were simple, their core content was very uniform, i.e. the overall change in physical condition before and after PL was not limited to thyroid disease.

Among the 41 people, there were 15 patients with hyperthyroidism, 2 patients with post-hyperthyroidism, 5 patients with hypothyroidism, 9 patients with thyroid nodules, 3 patients with thyroiditis, 3 patients with goitre, 1 patient with thyroid cyst, 1 patients with thyroid tumor, 1 patients with thyroid cancer and 1 patients with thyroid cancer sequelae. A total of 41 people were either healed or significantly improved by PL, with 100% effectiveness. The 100% effectiveness rate is doubted by a lot of people. I wondered why. However, after some consideration, it is better to be realistic. Because I am only presenting the random clinical cases received. However, "randomness" can reflect the statistics more realistically and reliably.

The randomness arises in that these cases are not written specifically for thyroid disease; the thyroid disease is only one of their multiple conditions that simply happened in many studies. It is a true reflection of the difference between a PL clinical trial and a general medical clinical trial: PL method aims at the patients, rather than a specific condition, which is more in line with the real situation. In fact, patients with chronic diseases usually have multiple conditions. It could raise the greater doubts about the effectiveness of PL in the face of patients of the different ages, genders, and medical conditions. In other words, anyone with a thyroid condition, regardless of their other conditions and physical status, would be clinically tested with the same PL method. It is the clinical randomization. The randomized clinical statistic of effectiveness is more reliable than the results of experiments based on a deliberately selected sample.

In contrast, clinical trials with medicine are restricted in their scope of application by the selection of eligible patients according to the pre-defined criteria. In other words, your medical condition and physical condition must fit into its prescribed paradigm before a particular drug or procedure can be used. Because drugs and procedures may have negative effects or be ineffective for different people and conditions. This paradigm facilitates bulk, streamlined diagnosis and treatment by doctors according to a recognized pattern. However, it is hugely restrictive for patients. Because it is difficult for a person to get sick according to the paradigm required by medicine, other pre-existing conditions and physical conditions can hardly meet the fixed model of medical treatment. Because medicine is targeted, it only hits the set target; it is not responsible for injuring the innocent part. However, PL is not a medicine, it has no negative effect, and its target is the cause of the condition, i.e. the blockage of the meridians, rather than the specific condition. All illnesses seem to be different, while there is the same cause: a blockage of the meridians. Therefore, PL is not only safe, natural, and environmentally friendly, but also simplifies the process. Besides, it is a natural movement simpler than Tai Chi or Yoga, rather than a medical treatment, so that it can be done by everyone with the highest effectiveness.

Some people may ask: your cases may come from people who had the effective treatment with PL, while you may do not know that people who have the effective treatment of PL do not send their report to you. In fact, it is exactly what I would want to know. I would like people who have done the required PL experiments without the effective treatment could send their reports to disprove my conclusions. However, I am often confronted with the reality: even those unbelievers always achieve the unexpected results of PL if they perform it seriously. You will see the similar cases below in the clinical discussion.

Another reason for the 100% effectiveness rate is that the base of study is currently too small. After all, I have only received about forty clinical reports. Certainly, I would like to receive more cases, more than 1,000 cases would be better. However, due to the constraints of the current human, material, and financial resources, I can only receive these cases at random, and this base number at least gives a start to doing this experiment. In fact, many patients with thyroid disease who had healed themselves by PL do not write about their clinical experiences. Because they were just patients without the responsibility or experience to write reports.

It is often seen as a miracle that PL experiment achieved these amazing results. In fact, it is absolutely a miracle. Over ten years of promoting PL, I have regarded the self-healing effect as the norm, and the countless practitioners of Paida have become accustomed to it. I think that it would be strange for its ineffectiveness if someone really insist PL attentively. If someone claims that they have conducted PL for several years without effectiveness. It will reveal that the intensity and duration of their PL was far from satisfactory upon the simple research. It can be concluded that they are not serious about PL. Because they do not really believe it. Anyone who does not have faith in PL will show up the sign in their clinical practice.

If you have doubts about the veracity of this report, do not force yourself to believe it. If you would like to judge it, you must first do the same experiment yourself. My mission is simply to collect and disseminate information that is beneficial to human health, which contains a little bit of divine revelation or a new knowledge, a new way of thinking. If you have lots of resistance in your mind to these clinical reports written by the ordinary people, which fails to reach the academic standards, you could regard them as a kind of folk tale that I have collected at random to entertain myself.

## 1. Overall results of PL:

41 people were treated with PL, 19 of them were healed and the other 22 of them were significantly improved.

Among the 41 people, 12 cases stopped the medication voluntarily, 1 case was forced to stop due to drug allergy and 1 case reduced drug dose.

Because most people were suffering from a combination of diseases, i.e. they all had two or more diseases, some of them even had 10 or more disease, through the implementation of PL, the thyroid disease and other diseases had been improved or were healed simultaneously, i.e. the various symptoms of the body were improved comprehensively after the meridians were unblocked.

## 2. The details of the various diseases are shown as below:

Among 15 people who suffered from hyperthyroidism, 7 people were healed and 8 people showed marked improvement, 6 of 15 people stopped taking their medication voluntarily, 1 people was forced to stop and 1 people reduced drug dose. Two people with post-hyperthyroidism were improved significantly.

A total of 5 people with hypothyroidism were improved significantly and stopped taking their medications voluntarily.

Among 9 people who suffered from thyroid nodules, 6 people were healed and 3 people were improved significantly.

Among 3 people with thyroiditis, 2 people were healed and 1 people was significantly improved. One of 3 people voluntarily stopped taking their medication.

Among 3 people with goitre, 1 people was healed and 2 people showed with the significant improvement.

One patient with a thyroid cyst and one patient with a thyroid tumor was healed.

One person with thyroid cancer was healed, who not only recovered completely but the removed thyroid gland regenerated healthfully.

One person who suffered from the sequelae of thyroid cancer had been improved significantly.

## 3. Location and time of PL:

Most PL friends mainly conduct PL of the body's generic parts, even the whole body, i.e. Paida of the overall body. Only three PL fellows were healed or significantly improved after Paida only one or two parts. The time taken to heal or improve significantly ranged from a few days, half a month, a few months to over a year for the differences in conditions and the intensity of PL, most people did not clearly describe it. However, many people have clearly described the time they persisted in PL, the statistics was compiled for your reference as below:

Nineteen people who have recovered from PL persisted for the following duration:

Four people persisted with PL over 3 years, 3 people persisted over 1 year, 6 people persisted for 6 months, 2 people persisted for 3 months, 1 person persisted for over 1 month. Two people dissolved their nodules and cysts after only 1 time of PL, another person did not specify the duration of their time spent on PL in their sharing.

Twenty-two people who have significant improvement from PL have persisted with it for the following duration:

One person persisted for about 3 years, 1 person for 2 years, 8 people for more than 1 year, 3 people for about 6 months, 1 person for about 4 months, 1 person for 3 weeks, 1 person for half a month and 3 people for about a week. One person only conducted 1 time of PL, and another 2 people did not share a specific time doing PL.

Although thyroid disease was contained in all cases discussed, it was the same of two cases as each had different complications. Therefore, two categories of the cases have only roughly divided, of which the efficacy was verified by Western-medically available indicators in Class I, and the changes in the thyroid tumor was visible in Class II, which crossed over each other. The cases are discussed basically in the order from simple inflammation to cancer.

# Chapter 2 Clinical Discussion of Thyroiditis, Hyperthyroidism, Hypothyroidism, and Thyroid Cancer

## 1-1 The self-healing path of chronic thyroiditis

Hello, Mr. Xiao!

I'm sorry for the delay answering your letter for which I was in Berlin for a few days this week! My story is probably the same situation that people suffer and heal from illnesses, and the various factors overlaying it are so complex. It is hard to explain all of the details in a few words. I can only share my actual situation with you. If there is something else you would like to add, please let me know.

Some days ago, while I casually flipped through Volume II of the *Huangdi Neijing*, I was surprised to find the last sentence in Chapter 71 of "The cold-evil" as: "When there is cold-evil in the heart and the lungs, the Qi stays in the two elbows; when there is cold-evil in the liver, Qi stays in the two armpits; when there is cold-evil in the spleen, the Qi stays in the two thighs; when there is cold-evil in the kidneys, the Qi stays in the two hollows of the knee. All these eight deficiencies are the chambers of the organs, where the vitality Qi passes and where the blood travels. The cold-evil Qi is bad for blood, which must not be retained. If it stays, the tendons and bones are injured, the organs cannot be bent or extended, which is referred to as contraction. I was so happy to read it, as if I had discovered a secret.

I would wish that you have happy travels in Japan!

Liu Lu To Bai

My story:

Since I was diagnosed with chronic thyroiditis (also known as Hashimoto's thyroiditis) caused by the immune system in 2007, as many people with the disease, I began a long journey of seeking medical help, which reflected on my illness and questioning the basis and methods of Western medicine. In fact, since 2006, I have been feeling a lot of obvious symptoms of discomfort, and when I went to my Western medicine family doctor for an examination, without finding anything. I thought that if I had received a simple de-stressing and adjustment of the imbalance in my body at that time, I would not have developed the so-called real disease later. However, the treating principle of Western medicine is to wait for organic pathology before treating it.

After receiving treatment with thyroid hormone tablets from Western medicine, I was told that I should take medication for the rest of my life to replenish the thyroid hormones because my thyroid gland could not produce adequately. After hearing the diagnosis, you can imagine that how frustrated I was. Moreover, the supplement of thyroid hormone tablets does not heal as it only relieves symptoms and deficiencies, and the treatment method is helpless for the periodic inflammation caused by the regular attack of the thyroid gland by the immune system. After learning about the principles of Western medicine, I began to look for Chinese medicine treatments. I agreed with the philosophy of the holistic nature of the human body, and felt that many modern illnesses are caused by the fact that we have been separated from nature for so long that we are no longer seen as an union of mind and body. It is about being differentiated, alienated, and functionalized. Of course, the knowledge of Chinese medicine is vast, which is not easily grasped by the ordinary people. It is also a long road to travel in the search for Chinese medicine.

Before I met PL, I was treated intermittently with acupuncture and Chinese herbs. Even though I was still taking hormone tablets, my blood tests were not stable. It was not until I went to the 18th PL workshop this year that I voluntarily gave up the hormone tablets and devoted myself to the nine days of PL. At the camp, I experienced a rare physical and mental pleasure and relaxation, and the painful crying in Paida pain was straight to the heart, which slowly opened and released the heart knots that were tightening up. Therefore, I had realized the deeper meaning behind the simple PL method. The self-health management approach mentioned in camp also puts the power of getting and treating illnesses in our own hands. If we do not take responsibility for ourselves, no doctor can really heal us. Heart knots or emotions, habits, diet, life management and others can be two gateways to health and illness.

After I came out of the workshop, I felt like I had been cleansed and I was able to keep moving again with ease and pleasure. For a long time, the habit of Zen jogging in the early morning at the workshop also became a habit in my daily life (Of course, I gave it up now that it dawns late and rains a lot here in winter). I could devote myself to my daily life by insisting the habit. Lajin is consistently done for 15 to 20 minutes per leg, Paida is done intermittently. I could do Paida exercises when I do not have spare time. People can have better effectiveness of twisting waist exercises after Zen jogging. Once I realized that I was going to catch a cold, I did 100 strokes of hitting wall exercises. As a result, I did not suffer the cold.

What is more pleasing is that I have not taken any thyroid hormone tablets since the beginning of July, my blood tests have been normal in three times of examination. My whole energy and condition are better than before. I never dreamed of it on my own. During the period of medication, the medication became part of daily life as a family routine. Currently, I know that we are a big storehouse of medicine and energy, where there are endless treasures to discover and use. If you are kind to it, then the feedback to you is endless.

--Liu Lu , 2011-12-17

The report gives a concise explanation on the thyroiditis treated by the western medicine and PL. It is also useful for us to discuss more cases later. She had many obvious symptoms a year prior to her diagnosis. However, the Western examination failed to find out anything wrong. There is simple reason: the principle of Western medicine shall wait for an organic lesion before confirming the diagnosis at which time the diagnosis is often more devastating. Because the treatment involves taking medication for life, long-term medication can further lead to more negative effects and complications.

PL workshop that she attended was not designed specifically for thyroid disease, it is random for every patient. How is PL diagnosed? HC are observing and experienced, without paying attention to the name of disease. Because all diseases are just different ways of manifesting meridian blockages. Apart from pain and sand toxin, which are the most common forms of HC showing the degree and location of meridian blockage, each person has different HC. For example, the author's HC is painful crying. Crying was the most typical form of HC for heart disease indicating that the real cause of her illness is depression. Therefore, she writes, "the painful crying in the pain of Paida went straight to the heart, slowly opening and releasing the heart knots that had been tightening. I came to understand the deeper meaning behind the simple PL method. We are all our own miracle doctors; it is the same as that we all destroy our own health. Heart knots or emotions, habits, diet, life management and others can be two gateways to health and disease." In other words, it's all determined by heart from emotions to habits. Disease and health are further determined.

Her experience at the workshop was a systematic PL of the whole body, with complementary mindfulness techniques as meditation, Zen jogging and three days of fasting. After attending this camp alone and going home with consistent PL, her thyroiditis was healed without any medication. I received another briefing from the author in 2018, she informed me that she has not taken any medication and her medical tests have been normal after PL.

## 1-2 My hyperthyroidism and insomnia healed by PL

Hello, Mr. Xiao:

I come from Rizhao, Shandong Province. I have been suffering from hyperthyroidism since April 201. I also suffer from insomnia. The doctor said that it is a chronic disease, and I may take western medicine for a few years, while the disease may not be completely healed in the end, that is, I have to recheck regularly after I am healed. When I heard that, it was like a blow to the head. Going to hospital became my daily routine, taking medication, picking up medication and having blood tests. Every time I came home from the hospital, I felt very depressed. I was so depressed. Who let themselves have this disease? After taking Western medicine for a while, my white blood cells decreased and the doctor told me to stop taking the medicine and switch to RICOTEN and vitamin B4, which increased my white blood cells, but my condition did not improve. My body's immunity dropped and I often had a high fever. I had switched to the Chinese herbal medicine - anti-hyperthyroid pills without any choice. I was re-examined once every two months, with the slow effect. I still had hope about it. During this period, the doctor recommended Iodine 131 treatment, I still insisted on taking the anti-hyperthyroid pills. At least, it would do less harm to my body. Sometimes, the pills got stuck in my throat and I did not want to swallow them. However, I have no other way, and just insist on it!

According to the progress of the review data, I would be almost healed by the end of the year. Finally, at the end of the year, the result of the review was almost the same as when I first got it! All the previous work was lost. I had also checked my liver function and it was damaged, I was experiencing a lack of desire to eat fatty foods and have nausea in November, I took some stomach medication for my uncomfortable stomach. According to my judgment, the damage to my liver function was not related to the use of anti-hyperthyroid pills. The poisoning of my liver function is mainly caused by eating something that I should not have eaten.

The doctor told me to stop all my hyperthyroidism medication, so that the burden of my liver can be released. I was crying again at this time, which was my lowest point, I was lying in a hospital bed, with the grieving, desperate and scared feelings. One time, I fainted during the intravenous transfusion.

After stopping the medication, one day at noon, my heart was beating fast, and I was not resting well. I asked my husband to bring me the medication. While he was adamant that he would not give it to me, saying that I must stop to take medication, the more you take, the worse your body become. What could be done? I said it in despair. My husband usually believes in Chinese medicine. He pondered for a while and said, "I read on the Internet that Paida can heal many diseases, we should try it on your disease! I really had no choice. Thus, I agreed to the suggestion. He patted my arm with his hand, the black bumps appeared where he patted me, I screamed in pain. After about 10 minutes, I took a break and tested my pulse. The pulse dropped from 95 to 79 beats per minute. It was amazing! I felt much better, my arms were relaxed and my whole body became calm. I was so happy that I slept comfortably for over two hours.

Since then, I have known about Mr. Xiao Hongci and PL. I have been watching your video lectures everyday to learn PL. gradually, my insomnia disappeared, and my body gained the energy, which increased my confidence. There were times when I cried from the pain during Paida. When I conducted Lajin, because I did not have a stretching bench, I used a chair. My tendons were soft, so I put weight on my feet and legs. I insisted on 15-20 minutes of Paida per leg at one time. Of course, I can conduct Lajin for 30 minutes per leg. I kept PL for 2.5 months and my body felt better, my heartburn and weakness disappeared, and my bowel movements became normal. At the beginning of April this year, I went to hospital to check my T3 and T4, and the lab results showed that they were normal. At that moment, I cried. I was so excited and moved - all of them was welled up in my throat.

Thank you, Mr. Xiao. Even though I know that the word "thanks" is too light, I am grateful to Mr. Xiao.

Best wishes: May Good people be safe and sound all their life!

--Tang Hong, June 28, 2013

Compared to the previous case, insomnia was also diagnosed in the case. In fact, insomnia is a symptom of depression and heart disease, as it is caused by the blockage of several meridians. Among them, the heart and pericardium meridians are paramount.. However, Western medicine can only address the symptoms, rather than the cause. Thus, "Visiting the hospital, taking pills, getting medication and having blood drawn for review became a routine."

Next, the negative effects of the medication took shape: a decrease in white blood cells. She changed her medication again, she suffered from the frequent fevers, and then changed to Chinese herbs until her liver function was impaired. She was hospitalized to treat her liver and stop her hyperthyroidism medication. However, nobody knew that she had a heart condition. Because the indicators were not enough to reach the organic pathology. The problem was that "One time I actually fainted when I had the intravenous transfusion." Fainting symptoms are a sign of a serious heart condition. Why do people with hyperthyroidism often have a tachycardia? if it's not heart disease? However, it is not enough to confirm a heart condition. What shall we do? It shall wait until there is a symptom.

Her husband gave her Paida for only ten minutes first, her pulse dropped from 95 to 79 per minute, which is the healing effect. How about the diagnosis? It was the black bruises that came out of her arms, which indicated blockage of the heart, pericardium, and lung meridians. What is the name of the disease? It does not matter! But it is certain that the result is certainly heart disease, depression, hyperthyroidism, and other illnesses. Because of the clinical experience, she has developed confidence in PL. The real healing started with a transformation in her heart. Because her heart decided to do PL. It was a choice that nobody could make for her.

"Therefore, I insisted on PL for two and a half months, my health improved, my heartburn and weakness disappeared, and my bowel movements became normal. At the beginning of April this year, I went to hospital to check my T3 and T4. The lab results were all normal." It is so simple and quick!

In fact, the main thing she healed herself of was depression, followed by heart disease, as two symptoms were verified by the bruises from three meridians of the heart, pericardium, and lungs. The symptoms of heart disease were also shown as fainting and tachycardia. However, heart disease is not diagnosed conclusively, and depression is even more difficult to diagnose, and all we can do is wait for the organic lesions to appear and use indicators to determine the name of the disease. Therefore, hyperthyroidism appeared. The doctor and the patient had been busy to heal it.

## 1-3 PL heals the eight-year hyperthyroidism and improves hot temper.

I am Ms. Zhou, live in the Golden Horse Community in Beibei District, Chongqing. I am a member of the Beibei Park Beat Group "Golden Horse Group" (It is the name given from Boss Cao).

In early August last year, Liu Qingbi from our community heard about Paida Group of Beibei Park in Lichuan and took us to the park and found the place where the group was active every night and saw that there were 30-40 people for Paida lively. Thus, I went to join Paida with the trying intention. It has been lasting for the half year so far.

I had suffered from hyperthyroidism for nearly eight years. My eyes were bulging out and I can not see clearly, it was too serious to be unable to close my upper and lower eyelids (lids) with photophobia. I had to wear sunscreen outside. It needs to spend RMB 700 to RMB 800 a month to control the deterioration of disease. After several months of Paida, I am completely off the medication and have a 70% reduction in my bulging eyes now, the vision of both eyes has been significantly improved no more photophobia.

PL has also improved my impatient and irritable personality. I was easy to get angry for the slightest thing in the past. My husband became my doormat. I have calm status and rarely get angry and quarrel now.

My health has been restored by PL. Thanks to PL method. The support and perseverance of our Beibei Park PL team for each other reflects a powerful positive energy!

At present, I keep Paida every day, so that I can be fit and healthy. Thank you so much!

-- Ms. Zhou, 2019.3.7

The external symptoms of the case become more obvious: bulging eyes, blurred vision, inability to close the eyelids, photophobia, and spending RMB 700 to RMB 800 per month to control the deterioration of condition. The eyes are so ill, which indicates the strong heart fire and the liver fire, it is known as the strong monarch fire and the ministerial fire in Chinese medicine, which indicated that the heart and liver meridians are blocked with the high temper. In depression, it is the irritable type. She said, "PL has also improved my impatient and irritable personality. I was easy to get angry for the slightest thing in the past. My husband became my doormat. I am calm and rarely get angry and quarrel now."

Why did her eye bulge improve by 70% after stopping the medication, her vision was improved significantly without photophobia? Because many symptoms stem from taking medication. When you take too much medicine, it is difficult to tell the original symptoms and the negative effects of the medicine. If you read more cases, you will find that many hyperthyroid patients suffer from liver damage after taking medication, which is the same as in the last case. There are many more later. Without the negative effects of the medication, the heart and liver meridians are unblocked by PL and it is easy to self-heal hyperthyroidism. Why was she able to stop the medication completely after a few months? Because mutual Paida can be done everyday in the PL group of Beibei Park, many people would share it everyday. Thus, the effect of mutual Paida and the spiritual resonance is better than doing Paida to herself, for which Boss Cao was also hosting the Paida.

## 1-4 Hyperthyroidism was healed and anxiety was significantly improved

Sharing from Collection Form of PL Case: Ms. Cui; Weihai, Shandong; Age: 38

Health condition and main health problems before PL: hyperthyroidism and anxiety.

Duration and frequency of practicing PL: Practiced PL for over 1 year, 1 time a day.

Duration of each Paida: 30-60 minutes.

PL process: Full body Paida, lasting Paida up to six hours. Conduct Lajin twice a day, once in the morning and once in the evening. One time for 20 minutes.

Physical condition after PL: Hyperthyroidism healed and anxiety had been significantly improved.

-- Ms. Cui September 2018

There is a case from the Collection Form of PL Case. It is brief information because it was filled out in form. However, the core message is obvious: her main condition is anxiety, i.e. heart disease. Once the heart, pericardium and liver meridians are opened and the mood gradually improves, the hyperthyroidism will heal itself. Moreover, she conducted Paida on her whole-body for a maximum duration of 6 hours and Lajin twice a day, and Lajin is effective in opening up the liver meridian. With the heart and liver meridians cleared, anxiety can be naturally improved, so that the self-healing of hyperthyroidism became almost a by-product, as the main symptom stems from the heart.

## 1-5 Hyperthyroidism antibodies were normalized by eight months of Lajin

I had all my hyperthyroid antibodies checked today and I had stopped the medication! I had stopped the medication for a week and my doctor told me to re-examine in 3 months in case it recurs.

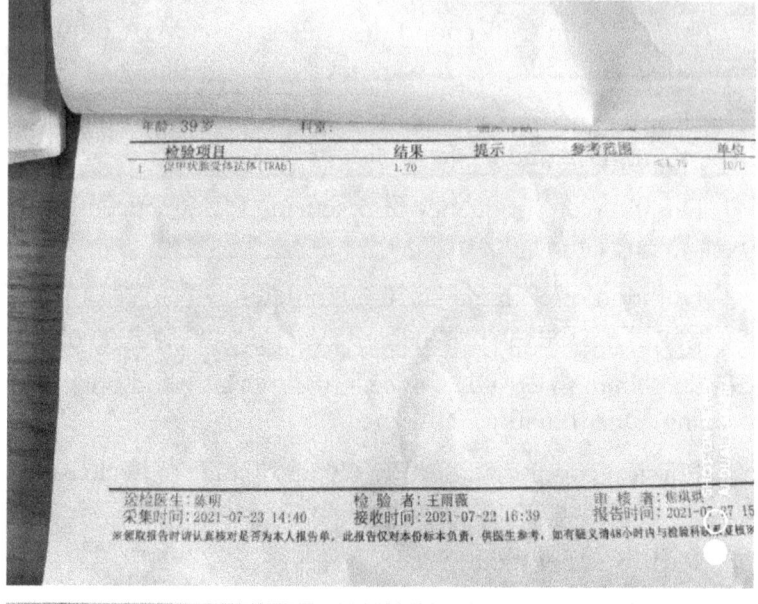

Y-

My hyperthyroidism was detected in July last year and it lasted for a whole year. I do usually Lajin frequently, Y-shape Lajin and lying Lajin basically everyday. I stretched half an hour; the upper leg is loaded with 3 Kg and the lower leg is loaded with 5.5 Kg for

25 to 30 minutes. I also insisted on moxibustion from neck to feet one hour each time.

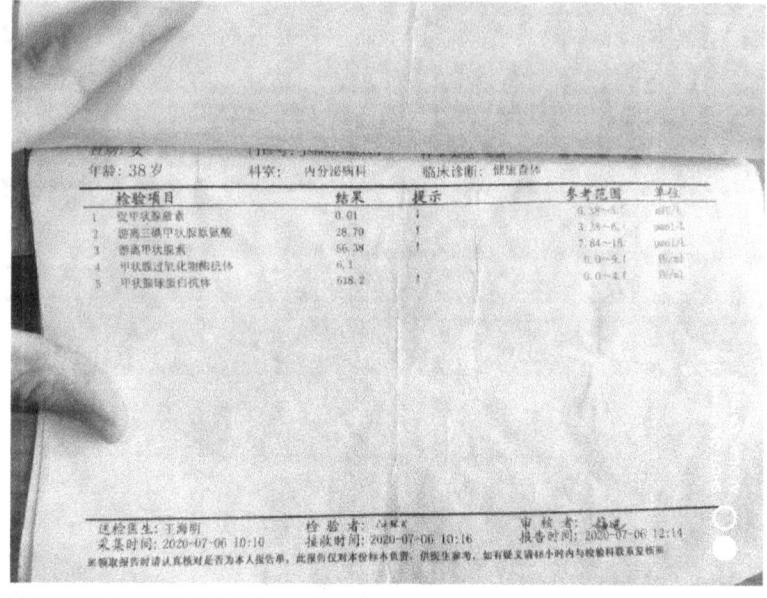

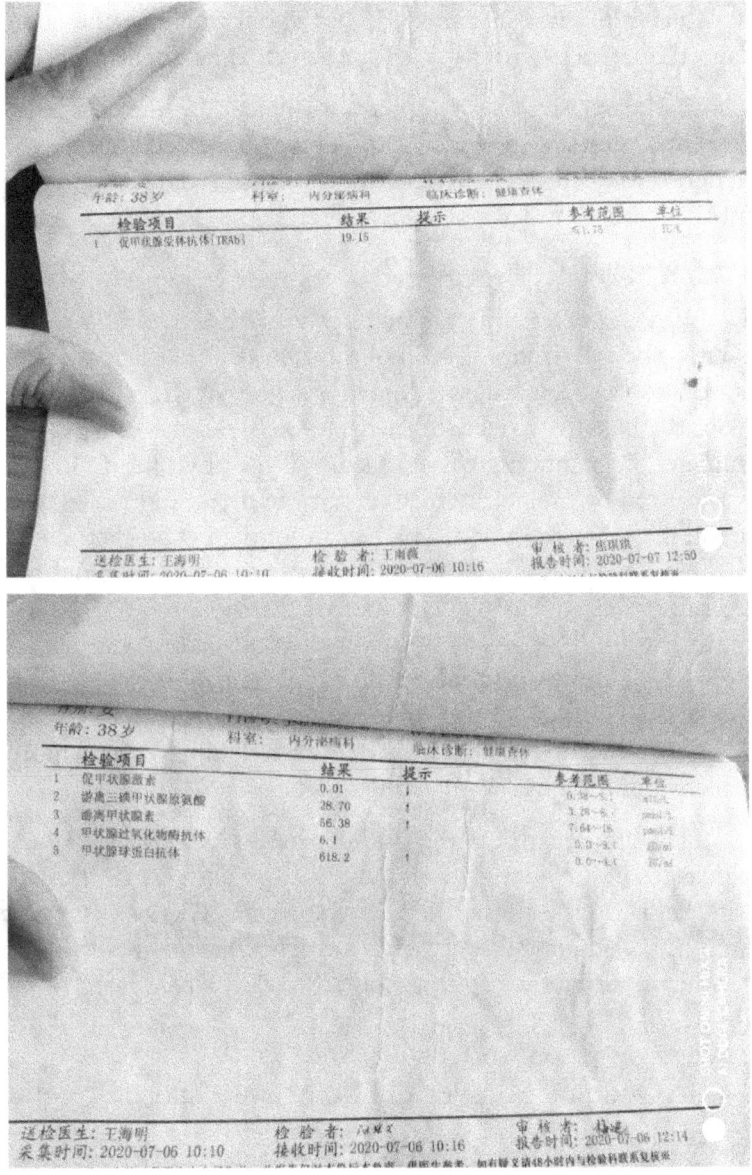

I also took medication, since I conducted Lajin on November 15th, last year, I changed the dose from 1 pill to 1/4 pill. At present, I have stopped taking medication for a week.

Although I am patting less, I can guarantee half an hour of face patting everyday. I still have a lung nodule at this check-up, which is as big as last year; I also have abnormal liver function caused by hyperthyroidism before, which is normal currently.

My heart used to beat exceptionally fast. However, it is currently normal.. In fact, all problems were caused by hyperthyroidism. My parents also do PL everyday, and my mother's fatty liver has been healed after the physical examination.

--Qingyu Youlan, 2021.7.29

Why did the main Lajin help to normalize the indicators? Firstly, she started doing Lajin 4 months after her diagnosis, she started to use Lajin after her diagnosis, so that she suffered less from the negative effects of medication. She thought that her impaired liver function was caused by hyperthyroidism. In fact, it was caused by the negative effects of the medication used to treat it and her negative mood. The heart meridian is blocked due to depression, and the heart meridian must result in the blockage of liver meridian. It can also be said that the monarch fire ignites the ministerial fire. Originally, the liver is wood nature and the heart is fire nature, and wood produces fire, so the liver is the upstream of the heart. Thirdly, she had the patience to moxibustion for one hour everyday, it was also worked. If it would have been more effective if one hour was used for Paida.

Her rapid heartbeat and nodules in her lungs indicate blockages in the heart and lung meridians. They are best treated with Paida on the elbow and the whole arm. The blockage of two meridians is the main cause of hyperthyroidism. If Paida is conducted properly, the lung nodules will dissipate faster.

## 1-6 Is Oedema all over the body only caused by the thyroid gland?

I am grateful to Mr. Zhang Shuangwen, I have been healed well at present! On June 20, 2016, I was so angry I was unable to pass stools in October, my weight suddenly increased from 57 Kg to more than 74.5 Kg, and my body was so swollen that I could not walk. I went to a hospital in Beijing to visit a Chinese medicine doctor and ate more than RMB 1,000 of medicine. But it did not really work, my friend introduced me to physiotherapy and spent more than RMB 3,000, it did not work after doing 9 laxatives.

I can only take laxatives to maintain a normal pool. I was referred by a friend to visit a famous Chinese doctor. After a month of medicine, I became better, but I was still swollen all over the body. I was told to go back and take the medication. The doctor also said that more than 90% of people have this disease, and it can not heal completely so the patient should take medication for life and have regular check-ups.

In June 2017, a friend of mine, Ms. Dong, introduced me to this PL group of Zhang Shuangwen. I saw the results of the family members in the group after Paida: their bodies got better. Under the guidance of Zhang Shuangwen, I went back to the Beijing hospital for a blood test one month after the whole-body Paida, and the results of the re-examination were that I was free of thyroid disease. The doctors were amazed when they read the medical report and surprised that how could it be possible!

After reading the report a month before and a month after, I was told to come back to hospital in six months for a check-up. After returning home, I patted different parts of my body everyday until the end of January this year, and I am still patting everyday, and I have lost weight from 74.5 Kg to 65 Kg now. I am grateful to Zhang Shuangwen for creating PL group.

--Shared by Ms. Liu; Collated by Volunteer Mo Fei; December 12, 2018

It is a typical case of heart-made illness. Anger was triggered the constipation and wild weight gain. It is blockage of the heart and lung meridians triggered by depression, while there is correlation between heart and the small intestine, as well as the lungs and the large intestine. In the appearance, that is, there are the mutual causes and effects, so that the large and small intestines are blocked, and constipation is further caused. Swelling of the entire body is obviously a blockage of the kidney and gallbladder meridians. It is judged from the symptoms. However, the diagnosis can be confirmed immediately by Paida on the general area. These meridians mentioned will produce bruises furiously. And, if you pat all the limbs again, you will probably be healed.

However, Western medicine confirm the diagnosis by biomarkers. "The various blood tests had costed more than RMB 2000. The final diagnosis was thyroid disease." What she tossed around for a whole year, from June 2016 to June 2017, a name of the disease and a lifelong regimen of medication was obtained. As she attended Mr. Zhang Shuangwen's PL group, "After a month of PL was conducted for her entire body, she went to the Beijing hospital for a blood test and re-examination, she was found to be free of thyroid disease. The doctors were amazed when they read the report and said, 'how was it possible?'." She would have been healed if she did Paida six months ago, or a week.

From these cases that have been discussed, the complications of hyperthyroidism vary, with the same causes broadly, i.e. they are all caused by poor mood, i.e. varying degrees of depression. It does not matter if you do not know the meridians, Paida of the whole body is certainly the right thing to heal the disease. Because all causes of disease cannot be separated from blocked meridians throughout the body. When the swelling goes down, it means that the gallbladder and kidney meridians have also been opened.

## 1-7 Therapeutic effect of high intraocular pressure and hyperthyroidism in an elderly German

Mr. Xiao: Hello!

I was working at my computer just now when I suddenly heard a sound of Paida in the garden downstairs behind me. I went to the window and saw that my neighbour, Mrs. Gertrudis, was patting intently in her garden.

I had taken her to your home a month earlier, the 70-year-old with hyperthyroidism and partial blindness in her eye vision accompanied by the increased eye pressure. She was worried about her eye condition. She had sought medical help everywhere, insisted on taking her medication and had regular check-ups. However, for the past two years, the results of each check-up had aggravated her worries, as her eye pressure had become higher over time. She had been frustrated and told me that she was afraid that she would go blind in the future.

About 3 months ago, I shared her with PL. Besides, at the last time, you went to her house to give her the "secret" in Germany. Since then she has been persisting with Paida on her arms and legs everyday, and adding an extra ten minutes of Paida for her eyes. Recently, she surprisingly told me with the results of her latest eye examination, which showed that her eye pressure had started to drop at the first time. In addition, her hyperthyroidism had almost disappeared, and she had stopped taking her medication. However, her eyes are too vital for her to stop the medication yet. From her joyful and hopeful look in her eyes, I believe that she would stop the medication completely soon.

She also shared her experiences with everyone around her. Every time we met, she would proudly tell me how many more people had been added to PL team under her influence and her fellows had achieved good results after Paida. She also took the time to write down her experiences and post them online for more people to share.

Currently, it is the height of summer in Paris where you are. I would hope that the little scene photographed will bring you a touch of comfort.

Xia'an

--Xue Xiaodan on 2012-7-27 in Duisburg, Germany

Hyperthyroidism and high intraocular pressure are different conditions in Western medicine, for which the different medicines are used. If you would find the cause by the further analysis, you will find that they are the same meridian blockage, the different symptoms in the body are just shown, mainly blockage of the heart, lung and liver meridians, and the liver meridian blockage is related to the application of medication. Interpreted in Western medical theory, it is a variety of inflammatory conditions caused by the overactive microglia. If you are involved in more various diseases, you will find that all inflammation, whether central or peripheral nerve inflammation, is caused by a blockage of the meridians. Therefore, the opening up the meridians can eliminate any kind of inflammation. It is especially true for three meridians of heart, lungs and pericardium.

The elderly German woman did Paida lightly with good effectiveness. Because she had not attended the workshop, it was difficult for her to pat the whole body. Otherwise, it would have been more effective. The author had sent a Paida video of the old man in the garden. The Germans are serious implementing Paida.

## 1-8 Daughter's thyroid antibodies were normalized after Paida

I came from Zhouwang mountain. It was also my first contact with PL. However, I do believe it. My daughters were not convinced that PL has so good effectiveness at first. When we spent more time together during the Chinese New Year, I did Paida for them, believe it or not, especially my second daughter, who had been taking Chinese herbs for almost a year after her thyroid cancer surgery. However, her thyroid antibodies were still high after doing moxibustion for more than half a year.

I did Paida for her when I had time around the Spring Festival. Because she was pregnant, I did not dare to use force. I had to consult with my experienced fellows for Paida, and their answers boosted my confidence.

At the first few days of the New year, she had another thyroid antibody test done in Tianjin and the antibodies were normal, except for the slightly high thyroxine, the high antibodies meant Joben's thyroiditis and the risk of recurrence.

-- Ms. Zhang, February 27, 2018

After almost a year of taking herbs and six months of moxibustion, her thyroid antibodies were still high. She only did Paida for her daughter a few times around Chinese New Year and her antibodies were normal in her reexamination. It means that the strength of Paida of the meridians is still deeper and more thorough. Of course, the herbs and moxibustion also played a role. If the daughter believes in it and integrates PL into her life, pats for each other and by herself, the effect will be sustainable. The mother and the foetus can benefit a lot from PL on the pregnant women.

## 1-9 Hyperthyroidism and lung nodules healed after six months of Paida

I came from Chongqing, with Internet name of Mother Tiger. On January 1, 2018, I still remembered clearly. At that time, as a middle-aged person, I suddenly experienced the pressure of having old parents and young babies. My 4-month-old child was hospitalized for bronchiolitis. My mother and my husband's father were hospitalized separately. Myy husband's mother while not hospitalized,   had diabetes combined with aortic sclerosis. Really, it was so stressful at that time.

My mother was diagnosed with hyperthyroidism in 2015 and lung nodules with suspected metastases in 2018, which scared me at the time. She was hospitalized for a month, and I was really tired out because I did not have time to take care of my mother even with the kids. Originally, hyperthyroidism could have been treated in hospital but do not know what happened to my mother. She had been eating western medicine in the Chongqing third-class hospital. After some time, she developed an itch on her body, her doctor suggested that she was not suitable to take that pill, and suggested her drinking Iodine 131, who said that my mother should be able to control the disease after drinking it once. I asked if there were any side effects, and the doctor said that there were fewer side effects than taking medicine, so that we had agreed.

At that time, the doctor was cautioned my mother about being in crowded spaces after drinking the medicine, I realized that this medicine is radioactive treatment, I was a little upset. A mineral water bottle cap of medicine cost roughly RMB 3000-

4000, she believed that the disease can be healed after drinking it. After 3 months, the indicators of my mum were not controlled. Thus, she sought the advice of doctor. It was recommended to continue to drink, the doctor said that my mum can keep taking Western medicine until hypothyroidism, for which lifelong medication shall be required, which is not as harmful as hyperthyroidism to the body. I was so dizzy listening to the advice of doctors. After treatment for about 1 year, my mother said that she needed to stop taking the medicine.

Because of her superstition, my mum felt that the hospital could not even heal her, she secretly ran behind my back to a temple above the Qijiang River in Chongqing, said that she could be healed there. I was so angry that I could not persuade her to come back. Because I knew that hyperthyroidism, the same as diabetes, had to be controlled. Otherwise, it would be complications. I had let her stay at the temple for 2 months without any choice and came back to check her indicators, which were even higher.

What shall we do? There is a good Chinese doctor nearby. Thus, we just tried Chinese medicine and took it for a year and a half. It was quite annoying to take Chinese medicine for a long time, and I do not know why my mum actually had better control with Chinese medicine than Western medicine. Although she was not healed, the indicators were close to the normal values.

However, after finding lung problems in 2018, she was hospitalized in another hospital and stopped Chinese medicine. Western medicine was used for treating her disease. During my mother's hospitalization, the doctor called me many times, the medicine cannot be used in a larger dose, my mother's white blood cells could not be stable, which could not be stable by the injection of white blood cells. I was anxious. This was useless, I knew that the injection of white blood cells was not good treatment for her. When my mother came back from the hospital, she even did not take any medicine, and then she went to the Chongqing third-class hospital to do a CT, said that there was a 1-cm spherical nodule on the lung, which was no progress from the film before hospitalization.

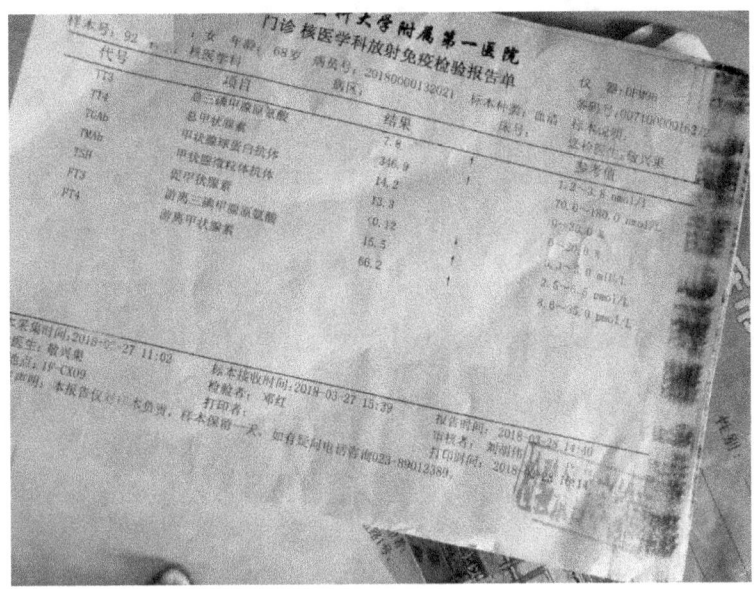

Examination report in March, 2018

I thought that the treatment of Western medicine can not be healed, the hyperthyroidism also turned over, with the higher indicators. I searched online for Chinese medicine methods, inadvertently searched PL. Afterwards, I found the customer service phone and WeChat, who gave me the WeChat account of Boss Cao from Chongqing Beibei, I also viewed Boss Cao's case on the Internet.

I thought that there was no other choice, the disease of the older could not be healed, I need to raise my child, my pressure can be imagined in the future. I contacted Boss Cao for the specific location and time, I ran to Beibei to learn PL. My family lives nearby Dadukou and it takes 4-5 hours to back and forth, so that I went there 2 times a week and conducted Paida for each other and by self. Boss Cao made up for Paida for me, Paida fellows were also helpful. Even it was pain really, I thought that there was still effect for I had a cold at the time, I went to the learning for several time. I believe Theory of PL, so that I introduced the specified method to my mother, and I began to help my mother to Paida.

After Paida on the body of my mother, the bruises came out fast and abundantly, it was amazing. As her first time of Paida, she patted the inside and outside of her arms, her back, and her front chest. My mum had never slept that long before, I was a little scared and checked on her in the middle of the night.

I taught her how to do Paida. Then she did Paida herself. She insisted on doing it everyday, except for eating and cooking, almost every morning, noon, and night. Moreover, she also did Lajin. Thus, she persisted with it for another half a year, and then asked her to do Standing meditation. After about 1 month, she also did PL diligently, accumulating 3 hours a day. Afterwards, she did a lung examination in July (and also did a test halfway through). The doctor said that the absorption was good, no mass almost was left, and she did not need to take any medication. She was normal.

Then a few days later, she had another hyperthyroidism test on the 13th of July. I thought that if she did not get well, she needed to just keep on the treatment. As the results would come out at 15:00 in the afternoon, my mother called me and said that the doctor said she was healed, I was so excited. I was afraid that there was a mistake, I asked my mother to come back quickly to show me if it was true. When I came back I got the medical report, all the indicators were within the normal range, I also felt amazed.

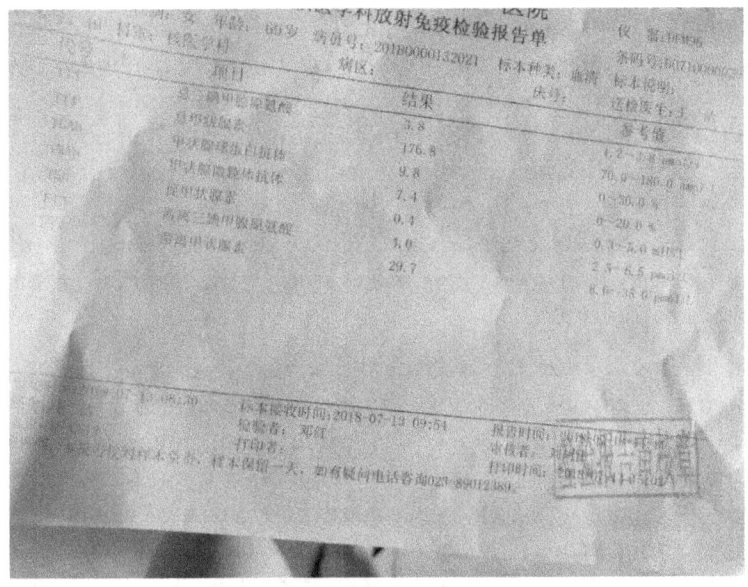

Results of the test on July 13, 2018

Therefore, I reported this result to Boss Cao at the first time, I am grateful that he has been working hard to do promotion of PL. There are quite a few persistent people who have gained health and admire my mum's persistence and perseverance.

--Mother Tiger, Chongqing mate, on July 15, 2018

We could figure out a clearer understanding of the Western medical mindset from the medical report. Compared to the subsequent PL, we naturally observe the phenomenon that only part of PL effectiveness is self-healing the primary condition such as hyperthyroidism, while the other part of the effectiveness is resolving the after-effects of the various medications in the earlier stage.

The author argues that hyperthyroidism was originally treatable in the hospital. However, I do not know what happened to my mother, who had been taking Western medicine at Chongqing third-class hospital and had developed an itch on her body for some time." She thought that this negative effect was an exception and there was really some kind of medicine that could heal hyperthyroidism. So, the doctor turned to suggest drinking iodine 131. My mum remained ineffective for 3 months of taking Western medicine. It is radioactive treatment with a huge negative effect! The doctor's advice was, "My mum can keep taking Western medicine until hypothyroidism, for which lifelong medication shall be required, which is not more harmful than hyperthyroidism to the body." So that it was the idea behind the treatment of Western medicine. We would learn a lot about the origin of hypothyroidism: it was caused by the medication for hyperthyroidism!

Because Western medicine did not work, she switched to take Chinese medicine. She took Chinese medicine for one and half year, which was better than Western medicine and made his indicators close to normal. However, a nodule was found in the lung, so she stopped taking Chinese medicine and switched to Western medicine. The negative effects were added: white blood cells were unstable. Then the injection of white blood cells was given, which had more negative effects in turn. The hyperthyroidism index was higher again. It is a typical medical clinical process. After nearly three years of treatment, the harm to the body can be imagined. What would have been the outcome if the treatment had continued?

It was at this point of desperation that she found Paida and was lucky enough to find Mr. Cao, a retired man who had been volunteering to promote Paida in the park for ten years. She learned PL here a few times before giving it to her mother to start. "When my mother did Lajin, the bruises came out fast and abundantly, it was amazing! For the first time, she patted the inside and outside of her arms, her back and her front chest." Note: She patted the six meridians (three Yang and three Yin meridians) of the hand, namely the heart, pericardium, lung, large intestine, small intestine and Tri-jiao, which were the most associated with hyperthyroidism and chest nodules. Moreover, at the front and back of the chest, the heart and lung organs are located. Paida method is the most effective in opening the severely blocked meridians of her mother, and its immediate effect can be seen in her HC. "As a result, my mother said she wanted to take a nap and slept from 18:00 pm to 8:00 am, without getting up." The long and restful sleep was the result of opening the heart and pericardium meridians and HC of heart disease. Her mother's poor sleep was diagnosed as a chronic blockage of the heart meridian. Her sleep was greatly improved and her strength was restored as a result of the long sleep. The damage to the heart and lungs stems mainly from the drugs and the mood.

Why did the mother heal so well Why did her hyperthyroidism and lung nodules resolve simultaneously? It really has to do with her mother's clinical efforts: "She kept PL everyday as usual, apart from eating and cooking, she did Lajin almost every morning, noon and night. Then she put up Lajin as well. She persisted for six months." It is rare for the average elderly person or patient to have such strong perseverance and spend so much time persisting in PL everyday. It showed that her own faith, determination, and perseverance played a decisive role. The clinical process is a simple repetition, as 0 and 1 in computer data, the Yin and Yang, the ups and downs. Your inner decision cannot be replaced by any family member or specialist.

Did PL heal the disease, or did her heart heal her?

## 1-10 Verification with facts: Paida is very effective for hypothyroidism!

On February 14, 2017, I gave myself a big gift on Valentine's Day through PL for over a year.

"No distortion, no distortion, no exaggeration, no exaggeration, speak with facts", these are a few words I particularly wanted to say after seeing this thyroid test report.

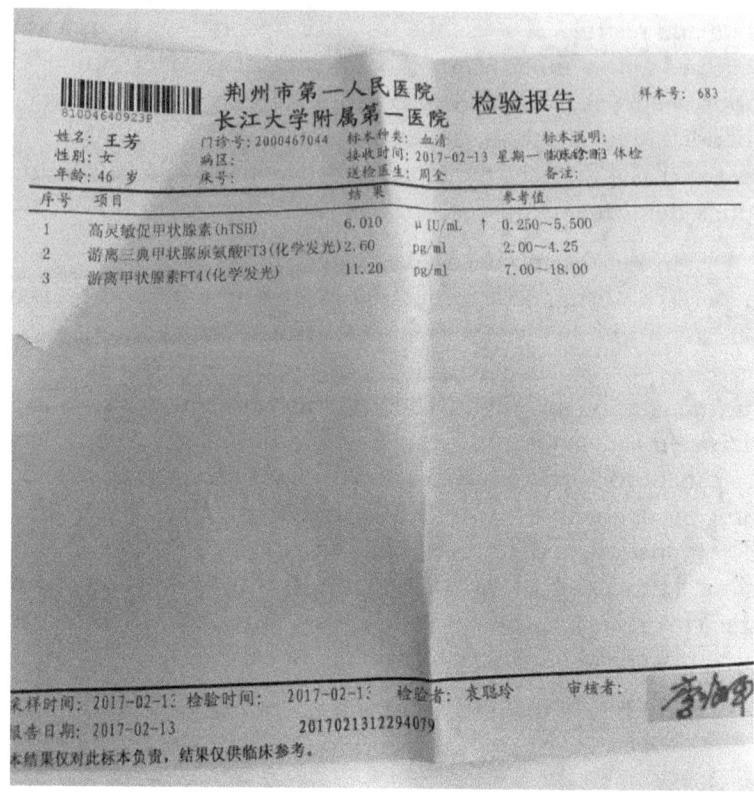

Here are my lab results sheets for November 2015.

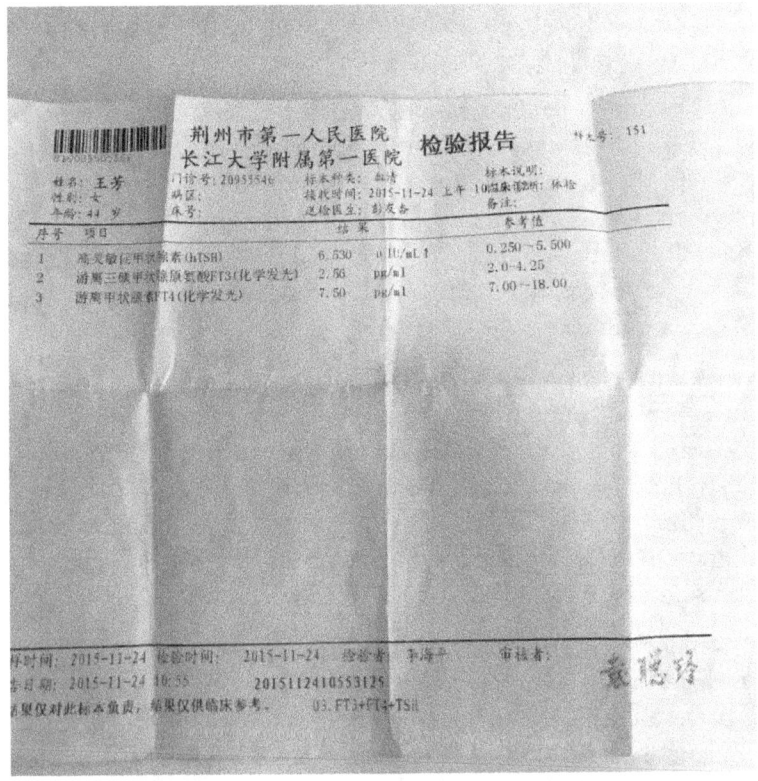

In 2000, I had hyperthyroidism and was prescribed to take Tabazol. I had never been to hospital before, except for giving birth, so I took the drug on the advice of the doctor, without thinking. A month later, I was in a coma with a high fever. When I was taken to hospital, I found that my haematopoietic function was hypothyroidism, caused by taking tapazol.

The doctor said that hypothyroidism had to be treated with medication for life. Because the body is sick, my mood was bad and low, my entire body was bloated, weak, and sensitive to the cold. From 2005 to 2009, I was hospitalized several times, my health becoming progressively worse.

People who may be physically ill are particularly concerned about the various ways to maintain health and heal illnesses. One day in June 2015, I came across PL on the Internet and saw that many people had been healed of many illnesses by Paida on their own, so I would have a try to get a better body!

I bought a Paida stick and started PL. It was a hot day and I was wearing short sleeves, so I had bruises on my arms and people thought that I was suffering from domestic violence and looked at me with pity. I did not care about it at that time, I just read Mr. Xiao's blog about patting the universal parts, so that I did Paida on my arms and legs many times, and wherever I was uncomfortable.

As for the symptoms of itchy eyes and hemorrhoid bleeding, the sore had been improved soon. The most surprising thing for me was a Paida of ringworm on the back of my neck that had been there for two years, its size was a dollar coin at the beginning and slowly getting a bit bigger. Anyone who has had eczema or ringworm knows that these things itch is harmful and every time you scratch until it bleeds, it does not relieve the itch.

Since it was on the back of my neck, I could not do it myself, so that I asked someone to do it for me. At the first time of Paida, it broke the skin and bled, so I thought it had cleared up. After a while it grew and I was a little disappointed. At the second time of continued Paida, the skin continued to break and bleed, after that I had moxibustion, I did not even know when it disappeared. I just remembered that when I was looking through the photos and it gave me a lot of confidence.

In November 2015, Mr. Yang brought me into our local PL group in Jingzhou - Apinea - and participated in a public service event promoting PL by Apinea to companies. Therefore, I became an organized person and was no longer a scatterbrain.

At the end of 2015, the eugenol that thyroid patients take was not available at all pharmacies at the time for some reason and people had to go to hospital to buy it, it was a hassle, so I thought that I am doing PL now. Why not try to stop taking the drugs?

As for taking the drugs, I had palpitations. In 2005, I took the liberty of stopping my medication for two months and then went back for a check-up and believed that the results would be more accurate. Am I a doctor?  At that time, I had whole body edema, my eyes were swollen and could not be opened, the calves could not walk and lifted, the doctor said: "Are you a doctor? I'm a doctor." I had to take my medication seriously for the rest of the day, except for one meal today when I came for a blood test. I was so scared that I did not dare to stop taking my medication.

However, it was different this time, I kept PL. At the end of November, I went for a triple-test of thyroid function, I started to stop taking the drug.

I completed a full-body Paida in December. When a lot of bruises came out in places where I had photographed many times. bruises are a kind of relief, all the illnesses had come out and bruises disappeared.

In March 2016, I started a second round of full-body Paida, and a lot of bruises came out. When the bruises disappeared, I kept patting again and again. I consulted Mr. Yang Weijie from Macau about the part of Paida for hypothyroidism. He answered me that apart from full-body Paida my whole body many times, I should also focus on patting my front, back and neck. I did as I was told and my body felt better, my hands and feet were not cold anymore, and my rhinitis had been improved. Afterwards, I even forgot about hypothyroidism.

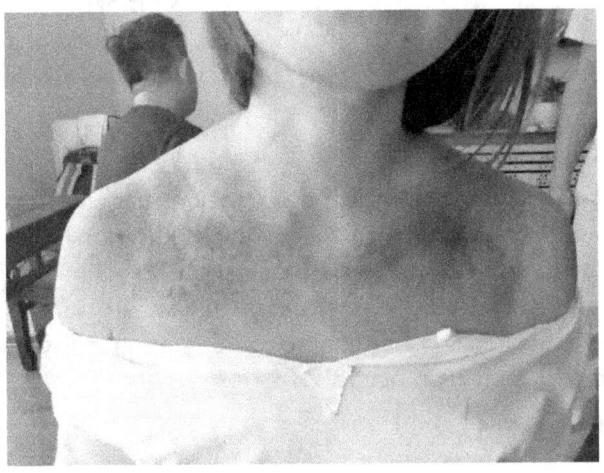

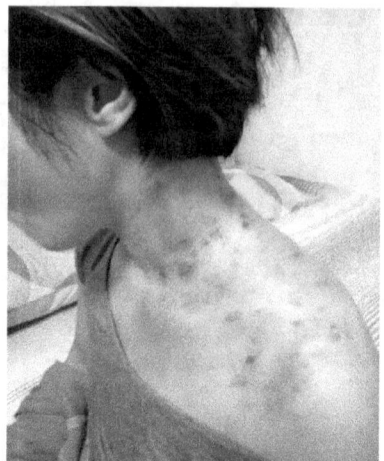

There are my photos of Paida in 2016.

In December 2016, I took part in the Spring Festival Gala held by Apinea Group, and I could not get into shape during rehearsals for stress. On December 31, I remembered it when I was talking to my good friend Zhang Rong, and I thought it must the onset of hypothyroidism, it was similar symptom, so I went home and looked for medicine. However, I did not have any drugs at home. I had to perform at the next day, so I did not have time to buy the drugs, so I did not take any drugs.

On the February 13, my son asked me to accompany him to hospital for a check-up, so I thought I would take a blood test myself since I was here. I believed that this result gave a strong answer.

Although the results of test were not within the normal range, I have not taken any medication for more than a year and my values became better than when I was taking medication. It broke the myth of the hospital that "hypothyroidism takes medicine for life". There is no disease in this world, it is only stasis and blockage. Just believe in PL and adhere to PL, so that everyone can take charge of their own health!

--Wang Fang    2017-2-16

From the previous case, we can know the thinking of certain western doctors, "Keep taking Western medicine until hypothyroidism, for which lifelong medication shall be required, which is not harmful than hyperthyroidism to the body." This case is the result of the implementation of the medical thinking. " In 2000, I had hyperthyroidism and the doctor prescribed tabazol for me to take. After a month, she went into a high fever coma, and was taken to hospital for a checkup.  Taking tabazol caused hematopoietic stagnation.  She was in the intensive care unit for a few days and nights to save her life-hyperthyroidism also turned into hypothyroidism, the doctor said hypothyroidism shall take medication for your entire life." In fact, it is not just hyperthyroidism that is treated, while in the process of treating hypertension, diabetes and many other conditions that have indicators, the indicators may improve or normalize because of the medication. However, more illnesses were shown, which can be even more damaging than the primary condition. In the first place, illness is a result of immune dysfunction, and treatment often results in worse immune function. As a result, the author struggled with the after-effects of her hyperthyroidism medication for over a decade, who was hospitalized several times.

After she learned to do Paida, she was able to improve her itchy eyes, bleeding haemorrhoids and ringworm after just a few Paida sessions on her limbs. Why was this seemingly blind Paida so effective? She later mentioned rhinitis, which was also a blockage in the lung meridian, and itchy eyes, which was a blockage in the liver and bile meridians. For example, there is correlation between lungs and the large intestine, so if the large intestine meridian is clear, the large intestine meridians must help the lung meridians to unblock, and vice versa; the liver and the gallbladder are also each other's exterior and interior, and any one of the two meridians will help to unblock the other. The lung meridian, large intestine meridian, liver meridian and gallbladder meridian are related to thyroid disease, which will help to improve the final thyroid disease, whether it is hyperthyroidism or hypothyroidism.

The recurrence of hypothyroidism she mentioned was clinically significant: "I could never get into shape during rehearsals due to stress. It was only when I was talking to my best friend Zhang on December 31, I remembered it when I was talking to my good friend Zhang Rong, and I thought it must the onset of hypothyroidism, it was similar symptom, so I went home and looked for medicine. However, I did not have any drugs at home. Thus, I had not took the drugs" In fact, they are HC, which can also be described as a relapse of an old illness, it is the same thing. "It was similar symptom" must refer to various symptoms. The cause of the symptoms is stress, which showed the direct effect of the disease of the mind on the disease of the body. Hyperthyroidism and hypothyroidism have the same meridian blockages as heart disease: the heart, lung and pericardium meridians, followed by the large intestine, small intestine and Tri-jiao meridian on the other side of the arm. In the previous case, why did her mother sleep for fourteen hours after the first time she did Lajin for her mother? Because she did Lajin for her mother's whole arm and front and back, taking in the meridians related to the heart, lungs and organs. Therefore, the good HC of "long sleep" was created. However, she did not open the cardiopulmonary meridians at the time. Because the pressure made the cardiopulmonary meridians more blocked, it caused symptoms of hypothyroidism that had not appeared for a long time. Unfortunately, she forgot to do Paida at that time, and Paida of elbows and the entire sides of the arms and the back of the hands will immediately resolve the symptoms. The illness also shows that its meridians have not been completely opened. She forgot to pat on it at the time, as patting on the elbow and the entire sides of the arm and back of the hand would have immediately resolved the symptoms. The offense also indicates that her meridians have not been completely opened.

"I have not taken any medication for over a year and I'm doing better than the values I've been taking, which shatters the nonsense of the hospital saying, 'hypothyroidism takes medication for life'. There is no disease in the world, only blockages and blockages." It seems that the result of stopping the medication and patting on it down simultaneously; without continuing to pat, the immunity remains abnormal and the medication can only replace the autoimmunity. However, the external medication will only further disable the autoimmune system. It seemed that stopping medication is the same as detoxification. The fact that she still had a lot of bruise after the second round of whole body Paida is a good indication that the residual toxicity of the previous medication is deep and numerous. If she kept patting her whole body, the strength and scope of Paida was not enough. She should have done Lajin along with Paida on her whole body again for a more complete effect on the meridians. Although indicators are available, it should still be a basic rule in the mind: the individual own physical and mental sensations are the most accurate. Indicators are meant to serve the person, rather than the master of the individual. If one relies too much on indicators and follows it, it is a disease of the heart. If the one usually PL consistently, the pain and the state of bruises is an accurate diagnosis of the degree of meridian blockage. If the individual conduct the regular and irregular mutual Paida vigorously, the diagnosis and self-healing is even better. If you have still any doubt about self-patting and mutual Paida, please refer to the next case.

## 1-11 Anterior heart pain, low white blood cells and hypothyroidism self-healed by stopping medication

I am a participant from Shanghai and I am 65 years old. I worked hard when I was young and had many problems: low white blood cells of 2.9; thyroid nodules and hypothyroidism; haematuria of 4+ with microscopic red blood cells of 20 or more; high uric acid; frequent irregular pain in the precordial region; migraine; fatty liver; atrophic gastritis and others.

Due to the chronic presence of these diseases, I had sought medical advice from various sources. Western doctors could not find the cause and prescribed medicines that was useless or even harmful. Even after taking Chinese medicine for a long time, I did not find out any improvement, but my gastritis got worse. In order to solve the problem for myself and my family, I studied everywhere, bought many books on Chinese medicine and health care, tried various methods, and looked for information on the Internet.

It seemed that I came across the information about PL on the Folk Chinese Medicine website and immediately went to buy the earliest version of the book *PL Self-healing* and read the blog of PL carefully, I could find the key to health. PL was performed intermittently and persisted for several years without major developments in my condition. However. When I got older, I often felt tired and weak for hypothyroidism and low white blood cells, and my haematuria got worse. Last winter, I had three colds and took about two weeks to recover each time, and PL was difficult to keep up.

When I saw the news of this workshop, I immediately signed up for it without telling my family and friends. I believed that maybe the self-healing method was the way that I should get fit.

In a few days, with the help of the instructors, I learned more about PL and experienced the power of the "Paida of overall body". The large number of black bruises was alarming. Although the pain of Paida was unbearable, it was a relief to discharge the toxins.

The clearing up of blood and Qi released my three worries. Firstly, I was worried about the dangers of stopping the daily medication for hypothyroidism. At present, it seems that there is no weakness or discomfort. Secondly, I was worried about whether or not I would be able to withstand the fasting.. Instead of being overwhelmed by the three days of restraint, I was able to complete activities such as Zen jogging and had the strength to help myself and my classmates with Paida. Thirdly, I was worried that I would not be able to bear the pain of Paida and what would happen after Paida of overall body. I could meditate on curing the lesions and enjoy the process.

Through a comprehensive and systematic PL, an individual's body and mind can relaxed. My feet relaxed, my heaviness was gone and my mental state improved. My sore throat and dull voice improved when I first joined the camp, especially on the evening of the sixth day when the pain in the precordial region of the heart basically stopped by Paida effect of the heart meridian for discharging bruise again. I could have the confidence to continue with PL method of self-healing in the future by participating in this camp, I could not only practice by myself, but also promote PL with my own experiences, more and more people will know and experience the miraculous power of self-healing.

I am grateful for the simple, effective and miraculous self-healing method, I am grateful to the three instructors who shared their way to teach us the correct way to maintain our health and help us to Paida vigorously, I have learned a lot of effective self-healing methods. Thanks, all the students, everyone's positive and serious attitude towards learning created an overwhelming positive energy that has contributed to everyone's health.

-- Ms. Zhu, April 17, 2014, Shanghai

The author listed ten diseases in the first paragraph and only skimmed the surface in the second paragraph: "Western doctors could not find the cause and prescribed medicines that was useless or even harmful." These conditions should be understood in this way: they are diseases that develop gradually over a long period of time while taking medication. For example, a decrease in thyroxine, i.e. hypothyroidism, may be the result of medication for hyperthyroidism. Other indicators mentioned, such as low white blood cells, blood urine 4+, high uric acid, fatty liver, gastritis, and others, were related to the long-term use of medication.

"PL was performed intermittently and persisted for several years without any major progression of the disease. When I got older, I often felt tired and weak for hypothyroidism and low white blood cells, and my hematuria got worse. It was difficult to persist with PL.." The quote reveals clinical information that can easily be overlooked and agreed with, assuming that the condition was exacerbated by aging. It is not the fact! The real reason is undoubtedly caused by the negative effects of long-term medication. In other words, the medication used for boosting her immunity and strength resulted in weakening her immunity and strength. It is a simple clinical fact that does not require to exaggerate. If you do not believe it yet, please look at the results of all the patients who took the same kind of medication as she did.

Another important observation: there are the older and frailer people, especially those whose illness is weakness, doing PL by themselves. It is not enough, so the effect is difficult to show. It is one of reasons that I repeatedly emphasize the mutual resonance of Paida. The author had to attend the workshop without notifying her family, which showed that they disagreed with her PL. They not only did not help her Paida, but they also prevented her from doing it. Is it love or hate? The improper knowledge could lead to a delusional spiritual decision. The desire to protect and love the person has the effect of attack and hate. It is easy to send your loved one to hospital and save their life! What is the outcome? Who would not be happy if hospitalization and medication healed the illness? If the condition gets worse after ten years or decades of treatment and countless medications, it seems that it is not only a physical illness, but an illness of the mind that is dominant. It is not normal to make the same mistake three times yet it is commonplace for the mistake to be made thirty or even three hundred times. The body's illness is a decision of the mind, and the purpose of the illness could be the improvement of the mind in turn.

It is the author's judgment that her fatigued and weakened condition was caused by hypothyroidism and low white blood cells. If we ask one more question: Is the root cause the hypothyroidism and low white blood cells? The medication is supposedly designed or intended to improve her symptoms. It is the paradox of countless medications, i.e., the medication taken exacerbates the symptoms, rather than reducing her symptoms. How can this diagnosis be verified? The results of her clinical experiment of Paida at the workshop and stopping the medication had the effect of eliminating her symptoms of weakness. The truth about the effect of the medication became clear; three days of fasting did not overwhelm her, she completed Zen jogging and other activities better, so the effect of fasting in detoxifying and clearing the meridians was clear. Although she worried about the pain of Paida and the consequences of bruises, she enjoyed the processes of these HC.

Looking at the improvement of her symptoms, her former fatigue and weakness became relaxed feet, her heaviness disappeared, and her mental state improved; the symptoms of sore throat and hoarseness at the time of entering camp improved; the pain in the precordial region basically stopped, which was the effect of Paida on the heart meridian again to produce bruise. The disappearance of weakness and heaviness is the result of opening the heart, pericardium and lung meridians; the improvement in symptoms of sore throat and hoarseness is the effect of the unblocking lung meridians; and the disappearance of pain in the precordial region is the result of the unblocking the heart and ppericardium meridians. The blockage of the heart, pericardium and lung meridians are all major causes of thyroid disease. In other words, the symptoms of thyroid disease are shown through symptoms such as weakness, heartache, and sore throat. However, just open the meridians throughout the body and the known and unknown symptoms will be naturally solved by PL. Nevertheless, it would have been difficult to achieve these results if she had taken her Paida at home without attending the workshop to Paida each other and supplemented by the instructor.

Therefore, she wrote, "In the course of a few days, with the help of the instructors, I learned more about PL and experienced the power of the 'Paida of overall body'. The large number of black bruises were alarming. Although the pain of Paida was unbearable, it was a relief to discharge the toxins." Where do these toxins come from? Most of them are medicinal toxins. The significance of PL is self-explanatory: it is not only necessary to open the many blockages in the meridians that developed into thyroid disease. It is also necessary to make great efforts to expel the medicinal toxins that are blocking the meridians. We certainly do not advise people to stop taking their medication blindly. However, we do advise you to PL well, and often pat each other. You could decide whether to stop the medication or not, and the pace of stopping shall be measured and discussed with your doctor in conjunction with PL.

## 1-12 Constipation, weakness, frequent urination, low thyroid, and prostatitis

I was fortunate to have the opportunity to fly from New York to Atlanta to attend the PL Self-Healing Course.

I am 72 years old and have stayed in the US for 38 years. I have operated garment factories, restaurants, laundries, and others. I have personally participated to work, my body suffer from many health problems, the most uncomfortable problem is constipation. I required laxatives everyday to, and I got up 3-4 times to urinate a night. I was also tired everyday for low thyroid. There are so many diseases in the body, while I can not find anything wrong in the hospital, I do not know how to treat it. Thus, I must keep taking medication. If there is no effect, I will change the medicine and take it. After six days of Paida, Lajin, Zen walking, Zen sleeping and fasting, I did my best and endured as much as I could. As the course was coming to an end, I benefited a lot. I stopped taking all drugs when I came to the course. On the fourth day, I passed stools without taking any laxatives. Besides, I also stopped taking thyroid and prostate medication. Even after taking thyroid medication, I had less energy all day. However, after three days of abstinence from medication and fasting, I felt better and less tired. In the past, I felt weak to urinate and I always felt that urine was not finished, while I feel better to urinate at present. I used to get up 3-4 times at night even with medication in the past. At present, the number of getting up at night without medication has been reduced to 2 times, which is really unexpected.

I have had a great feeling in the past seven days, and I have gained a lot. My outlook on life has changed, I should have a loving and supportive heart towards others, and I should be grateful to my parents and siblings, and I should be sorry and grateful to my body that I have suffered so many diseases from working industriously over the past few decades. I am even more grateful to Mr. Xiao for helping us to talk about self-healing therapy. How to do Paida on the different parts of the body with love, so that bruises can come out. Paida can stop until the black and purple bruises turn red. Lajin should be endured with pain and numbness. We shall persist with Paida twice a day, and achieve the better effectiveness with Zen jogging and fasting. I am also grateful to Ms. Ji Ying and Ms. Liu Rong, who kept telling us how to do PL, and even helped the elderly people personally. I am sincerely grateful and thankful.

-- The participant from the First Atlanta Camp Zhang Wenhuang, 2011-4-2

As the previous example, most illnesses of the author in this case were caused by taking medication. "There are so many diseases in the body, while I can not find anything wrong in the hospital, and I do not know how to treat it, so I have to keep taking medication. If there is no effect, I will change the medicine and take it." This passage shows a paradox that people take for granted: Why do an individual keep taking and change medication when no disease can be detected?

Clearly, the illness is clearly felt by the patient, while the doctor cannot find out the cause. How can you heal a disease if you do not know the cause? It does not matter, just treat it as usual! It means suppressing the symptoms with medication. However, it obviously has cost, there is the endless stream of negative effects, that is, new diseases are created, which is healed by other drugs. As for hypothyroidism mentioned above, it seemed that taking medication will not restore the thyroid function, it will only further lose this function. Weakness and constipation are common symptoms in many patients with thyroid diseases. From the perspective of meridian, they manifest themselves in the meridians on two sides of arms. Weakness is a symptom for blockage of the heart, pericardium and lung meridians, which is on the inner side of the arm; constipation is a symptom for blockage of the large intestine, small intestine and Tri-jiao meridian, which are on the outside of the arm. Therefore, you must pat your arms well in all directions, the bruises can come out. It shall be patted again after the bruises are gone. For example, after Paida of one arm for 2 hours, it shall repeat several times. You will be delighted with the effectiveness. It is used for the legs with the same method.

At the camp, we only conducted Paida once from head to toe, so we only learned to do PL, obviously it is not enough time to get rid of all the illnesses at once, while it was a good start. The results will be even better if we continue to keep patting ourselves at home. As for the effect of medicine, he has verified it with the clinical experiment: "On the fourth day, I defecated without taking any laxatives, I also stopped taking thyroid and prostate medication. Even after taking the thyroid medication, I had less energy all day. However, after three days of abstinence from medication and fasting, I felt better and less tired. In the past, I felt weak to urinate and I always felt that the urine was not finished, while I feel better to urinate at present. I used to get up 3-4 times at night even with medication in the past. At present, the times of getting up at night have been reduced to 2 times without medication, which is really unexpected."

In fact, another participant in this workshop had more incredible results when he stopped taking his medication. His name is Qian Xingge, a retired university professor. He had been taking prostate medication for ten years, who was awake up 4-5 times a night on the medication. After the first day of PL, he had a miraculous effect and slept until dawn without getting up again at the end of the seven-day camp. His blood pressure was barely 130/85 after 10 years of taking anti-hypertensive medication and dropped to 120/70 after he stopped taking drugs. His blood sugar was high without any medication, it was easier to heal himself, which was dropping from 204 to 108 (diabetes is over 100 in the US standard). You can read Professor Qian's case sharing in *Clinical of PL Report on Hypertension.*

Although the body has been improved, the most profound change of author is in his mind. He writes, "My outlook towards living has changed, I should have a loving and supportive heart towards others, I should be grateful to my parents and siblings. I should be sorry and grateful to my body."

## 1-13 Improvement of hypertension, heart disease, diabetes, and hypothyroidism after one year of PL

This report is characterized by a clear account of the history of the disease, the history of medication taken and the clinical course of medication reduction and discontinuation after PL. It is helpful in our understanding of the etiology of the illness and the outcome of the healing process. It can conclude that her medical history is the history of taking medication to increase her illness.

Her initial illness was insomnia. When she was diagnosed with PL method, it was a blockage of the heart meridian and pericardial meridian, i.e. a symptom of anxiety and heart disease. At first, she took Chinese medicine, while it was ineffective, then she took Western medicine. If she could not sleep, she added one tablet and then another, and the dose of drug became larger, while it was still ineffective. Thus, the doctor injected intravenous "sleep-strengthening solution" directly. These drugs were harmful to the heart and brain, so the negative effects accumulated into "Ménière's disease", which is still the result of the blockage of the related heart and brain-meridian. In 1992, she developed hyperthyroidism, and had surgery with 15 stitches in 1994, leaving her with the sequelae of hypothyroidism, she was required to take "Eugenol" for the rest of her life. It is another case of hypothyroidism resulting from the treatment of hyperthyroidism.

As with previous writer, she thought that she developed a series of new diseases for her age: hypertension, coronary heart disease, diabetes, stomach ulcers and herniated discs. How can a normal person get so many diseases with age? Obviously, it is the result of long-term medication. If you agree with the diagnosis of PL method, you will know that so many different conditions with different names are complications of heart disease, some of them can even be directly called symptoms of heart disease, such as hypertension, Ménière's syndrome, diabetes and hyperthyroidism. Because they are all conditions evolving from blockages in the heart, pericardial and lung meridians. The simple diagnosis is not agreed to Western doctors for its absurdity, but I am also afraid that Chinese doctors do not agree with it.

However, the author's clinical experiments with PL prove that it is just simple. Her Paida process is also a natural process of reducing and stopping the medication. Because the negative effects are greatly reduced by stopping the medication, PL is effective. Otherwise, "I take a lot of medications everyday. Sometimes, I was so confused that I did not remember the specific medications taken. There are a lot of Chinese and Western medicines." Because diabetes is given with insulin and medication, there is a burning pain in the cortex of the body. The doctor said that it is a complication of diabetes, neuropathy, and take another kind of medicine to heal the disease. In the chaos of so many diseases and medicines, how did she get it through?

She started specializing in patting on the generic areas one week. It is my favourite way to start a game. It is like playing chess with an opening move. Because Paida on the universal area is a comprehensive diagnosis of which meridians are blocking. Because the heart and pericardium meridians are patted first, it sets the tone for the whole-body meridians. The official of the sovereign has acted, which is the same as giving an order to the whole country. Moreover, Paida of the general area is also equivalent to a mini whole-body Paida. She saw" the results on the current day and felt relaxed all over, the more she did Paida, the happier she was. After a week, she stopped all the medication for blood pressure and heart disease, every indicator was normal."

Why did she have such good results? It is related to the significance of my talk above about the heart and pericardium meridians. Please look at her Paida clinic: "I started PL on February 12, 2018. It felt good to Paida on the elbow and the whole inner side of my arm, I was delighted and comfortable in my heart and happy to have such feelings." The area is located on the heart, pericardium and lung meridians. Blockage of three meridians is the root cause of heart disease, hypertension, diabetes and thyroid disease. Whether it is hypertension or low blood pressure, hyperthyroidism or hypothyroidism, hypoglycemia or hyperglycemia, Paida on the above areas will be effective. It could be more effective than the medicines taken.

"I started Paida on the general area for one week, then I started Paida on inner and outer legs and the popliteal fossa, and felt relaxed and refreshed all over." It's not a complicated area. Why did the same people who started Paida not have the same results as her? Let's look at her Paida method: "I did Paida twice a day on 4 parts, 2 parts each time. It takes about an hour and 30 minutes for the bruises to come out, and then I keep patting until the bruises is flat and dispersed. At night, I also did Paida on two parts for one and half hour." It means Paida on one area for at least 45 minutes, and keep Paida until the bruises dissipate. Do you have her patience and time to do Paida? It's easy to do Paida. However, it is not easy to do Paida attentively.

Besides, "At the other time, I did Paida at every opportunity. A scraping plate was always carried in my bag when I went out. I did Paida everywhere I went and shared it with others. Later, it was Paida of overall body, Paida was done on the whole body." In addition to Paida, she started Lajin in May, "Lajin was conducted in the morning and evening, as well as an hour after lunch, while taking a break for lunch." It is evident that her PL are beyond the reach of the average person. Because she did PL with her heart. The heart determines everything!

Her clinical summary of stopping the medication is shown as below: "At the beginning, I did not withdraw all the medication at once. When I did not feel unwell, I basically forgot to take the medication. Later, I did not get dizzy without the medication, I did not have any tightness in my heart or angina, and I did not feel uncomfortable. My hypothyroidism resulted in my hands shaking.. If my hypothyroidism onset, my whole body would get weak and tender. However, I was 90% after Paida. Therefore, I withdrew and stopped taking my anti-hypertensive medication, heart medication and eugenol." It shows that the criteria shall follow the sense of feeling. However, there are also people who feel well, while they are afraid to stop taking their medication. There are many cases in hypertension where they take anti-hypertensive medication even when they are normal, who will finally develop into dizzy symptom: hypotension!

She even stopped the insulin, and her medication was reduced to just 0.25 grams of metformin. It seemed that she is not blind at all, and she tested the related indicators to monitor her condition. In general, she uses her own feelings as the focus and takes the indicator measurements as a reference. Because she had many and severe illnesses, hypothyroidism was not even outstanding among them, especially after the symptoms of shaking hands and weakness disappeared, the memory of the illness and the associated medication faded.

Throughout her self-healing and medication withdrawal process, you will notice that she had a good start to PL by concentrating on the elbow and the whole arm, which opened the three most important meridians - the heart, lung and ppericardium meridians, and laid the foundation for unblocking other meridians throughout the body. Because above three meridians are directly related to all diseases. It can be said that the names of the different disease are just different ways of expressing the blockage of these meridians. Based Paida of the general area, and combined with PL of the whole body, the whole body meridians are unblocking. When the meridians are unblocking, the flow of Qi can be smooth, for which Qi is the most natural medicine of body, the repair and expelling waste are automatically completed, so that the diagnosis and treatment are completed simultaneously. It is so-called self-healing!

What is her masterpiece? It is just her faith and patience. The real healer is her mind! Many people have more knowledge and learning than her, while it is the knowledge that misleads them into a path that harms them. False knowledge and negative emotions are at the level of the mind, and knowledge and emotions can be changed. You shall decide it by yourself. If you change your mind, you will naturally change your body. Because the mind is the true master.

# 1-14 Why did I stop all my medication? -- Thoughts about the first Anniversary of PL

By chance, it has been almost a year since I first encountered PL. It has been one of the most transformative years for me physically and mentally, as well as pain and pleasure, PL is one of the most unique routines that I have followed in my many years of seeking medical advice, its appearance really changed my profound understanding of life and health.

**Reflection**

Looking back on the ups and downs of my life, perhaps I was tired of running around, focused on gains and losses, loved to save face, loved to show off, loved to lose my temper, in short, I wanted a lot and gave up too little. The psychological imbalance caused by physical imbalance, coupled with long-term overload of work pressure has not been adjusted and released in time, I have just passed the year of confusion is already riddled with many diseases.

In the past. When there was a problem with the body, I would go to hospital. Meanwhile, I blindly followed the doctor's treatment of my body. In 2000, I had an appendectomy for an acute attack of chronic appendicitis due to overwork and in 2007, I had to have my entire left ovary removed due to an 8.6 cm ovarian cyst (fortunately, the pathology was benign). In 2003, a physical examination revealed Hashimoto's thyroiditis, myometritis and endometriosis (a difficult gynecological condition). Speaking of these diseases, it is really an unbearable experience to look back on. Every time I had my period, it was like a day of disaster and the pain was unbearable. Sometimes I could not walk or get out of bed for the huge pain, or even roll around and vomit, and I spent one-third of each month in pain.

Since 2008, I have been suffering from lobar breast enlargement, fibroids, hyperlipidemia, hypertension, and diabetes. When I suffered from many complex diseases, for a while I really could not resist, I was busy running among the major hospitals in Shanghai. Do I have to deal with the hospital everyday for the rest of my life? When would I stop to take all these pills? I even felt that death was not far away from me, while I was helpless in the face of my own body.

Two years ago, I had a very bad attack of cervical spondylosis, I could barely hold my head up, and I had dizzying headaches everyday. I went to hospital and spent several thousand yuan on MRI, acupuncture and physiotherapy. However, nothing can be helped. I was recommended moxibustion, acupuncture, cupping and other methods, which provided some relief, rather than complete healing. However, a simple moxibustion accidentally healed my years of dysmenorrhea.

In 2010, I met a 20-year-old waitress at a moxibustion health centre who said her teacher had healed her dysmenorrhea with moxibustion. I asked her to try it at the time with a glimmer of hope. However, my years of dysmenorrhea was healed by a 2-hour session I had no onset again since then.

This experience completely overturned my views on the so-called formal hospitals and expert professors. I believe that the people have their own masters. Since then, I started to focus on ecological health treatment, i.e. abandoning medication and focusing on the external treatment and food therapy. The results were obvious: my blood lipids, blood pressure and fatty liver were all effectively controlled, and my weight returned to normal. I met PL again a year later and slowly, I felt a new energy in my little heart and a new energy in my little universe.

### Encounter

On 8:00 pm, December 24, 2011, a programme on health and wellness came to my attention by chance. An old lady in her 60s was introducing the details of Paida, so I lifted my arms and started PL as the same rhythm on TV. My wrists were sprouting little purple bumps within five minutes. I was so shocked that I asked my husband to give me a try when the TV was still showing the Paida method of the Weizhong acupoint. I felt that this method was amazing. When I thought about it calmly, Paida may be one of the methods of health care, just like Skin scraping therapy or moxibustion.

The next morning at work, I lifted my arm to show my colleague with the results. Coincidentally, she also held out her arm and it was even more purple than mine. We said that we did Lajin last night, she had experienced it at a friend's party on Christmas Eve. She had brought along a copy of PL *Self-Healing Manual* signed by Xiao Hongci. The first chapter of the booklet describes the five criteria of the self-healing method: Effectiveness, simplicity of method, safety of implementation, broad spectrum of treatment, and self-implementation. Its characteristics are derived from the Huangdi Neijing, which states that the heart is the top priority, focus on the main external treatment, the body should be supplemented by food therapy and final medicine. If it is the case, everyone can become a miracle doctor. I did not stop for a minute to read it three times. PL may be the last straw in my life, I must try it. It's so simple and easy, at your fingertips, it takes no effort to get it.

**Attempt**

According to this booklet, I started to practice Paida at home everyday. Meanwhile, I checked the Internet everyday for video materials and cases shared by blog of Mr. Xiao. Due to a lack of Qi and blood, I was very slow in getting bruises from the general area at the beginning. During the first few days, I felt very tired, and it was the winter season, so that I could easily catch a cold after Paida. I turned on the bathroom fan, sat on the flush toilet lid, and soak my feet by the electric heated foot soaking bucket and patting on my elbows, knees, and others. My whole body warmed up and a lot of bruises came out soon.

Every time the bruises come out, I feel a sense of accomplishment, just like when the Eighth Route Army fought and eliminated Japanese enemy one by one, occupied the favorable terrain, concentrated firepower to take a high ground, until the enemies were killed and completely surrendered. After continuous Paida of overall body for a month, I inadvertently found that my sleep quality had improved, slept peacefully, and my heart-beating was also steady (in the past, I had been flustered, I could not sleep well at night, and got up many times at night), I was convinced that Paida was working.

Meanwhile, I acted at good opportunity and bought a stretching bench from Taobao. It is a long square stool that is less than one meter square, with a wooden stick in front of it. I muttered to myself. The first time, I went on the bench, I only lasted for three minutes before I was too sore and swollen to do it. I could not flatten my legs that one side was high and the other was low. I could not put my right arm down (I had scapulohumeral periarthritis in my right hand). At this point, I realized that I had to take my time there was always a process of adaptation, so I made up my mind to increase my stretching time by one minute everyday. After two months, I started to follow the information about the camp on Xiao Hongci's blog to get a better grasp of PL's techniques and mindfulness and achieve the healing effect.

**Doubts**

It is same as all Paida fellows, I was able to persist on the daily Paida, but I always had a few questions in my mind: Are the articles on Mr. Xiao's blog true or not? Are the results amazing? I have diabetes without bad symptom. Although I did not take any medication, my blood sugar indicator did not improve significantly after a month of PL. It was always unstable, maybe what PL solved was just a symptom of the condition. I wanted to go to a workshop, while I was afraid that I would run into a money scam. After all, it costs a lot of money to attend a workshop. I searched through the various channels, called, and wrote to real friends to find out the real effect of PL. Until those who had come out of the camp and had achieved certain results told me personally that the method really worked, then I made up my mind to go to the camp in Yangzhou.

**Experience**

From February 25 to March 2, 2012, I attended the first PL 7-day course in Yangzhou. I was fortunate to meet nearly 100 Paida fellows from all over the world, as well as fellow Chinese from Taiwan and Canada. The oldest was over eighty years old and the youngest was only seven years old, while simultaneously feeling firsthand the strong warmth and aura of an extraordinary large group. The legendary Mr. Xiao attended throughout the event, his trademark goatee giving him an air of Taoism and immortality. His lectures were concise and easy to understand. He was always available to answer questions from the participants.

The most touching part of the camp was Mr. Xiao's mother, an old woman who was nearly 80 years old, a demonstrator of standard movements lying on a stretching bench, a Zen jogging leader who always came first on rainy and snowy mornings, and a volunteer who silently dedicated herself in the workshop. I was also impressed by the volunteer coach in the same group, Mr. Yuan, who felt like a father to take care of us. Because he patted the students everyday, his hands were almost all broken and bleeding, with a lot of Band-Aid tape on his fingers, which was really a heartache.

There are moving stories everyday in camp. A seven-year-old boy from Henan Province, Xiao Yuantong, was left with the after-effects of a high fever and excessive use of antibiotics in hospital at three years old, which resulted in muscle atrophy in his two legs. His parents searched the major hospitals in China to no avail before coming to the camp to report their last hope. At every time of Paida, his heartbreaking cries resounded throughout the 100-metre hall. I witnessed this child being helped up and down the stairs by his parents on his first day at the camp. After four or five days later, he was walking happily on his own, and the parents always had mixed feelings on their faces.

There is also an old couple from Beijing who are nearly eighty years old, the old man said that his son was filial to everyone and bought a round-trip train ticket to let the old couple come to Yangzhou to travel. While he did not expect it to be an extraordinary trip, their son was afraid that the elder would not accept it and did not directly tell them the truth. He did not expect that this trip was worthwhile, the quality of life of the old man in his later years was guaranteed, and the old couple finally understood his son's good intentions.

Li Ke, a thirteen-year-old girl from Suzhou, came to the camp alone, taking serious notes everyday and reported to her mother everyday, wrote and tweeted about her experiences. She travelled around at a young age, learned self-care and health management methods from a young age.

Thirty-nine-year-old cancer patient Ms. Hongbo, accompanied by her husband, attended the camp for the second time. She said she had just married and had come here for her honeymoon. The camp had given her hope for survival. The camp not only taught me PL techniques and mental cultivation methods, but also taught me an optimistic attitude towards life. Many participants were in tears at the sharing session before left. I suddenly felt a sense of rebirth when I left the camp.

**Fasting**

Fasting is a difficult and intimidating process. I did think so in the past. After coming to the Yangzhou camp, through the patient guidance of Mr. Xiao and the coaches, I was able to dispel my original worries and had a sense of trust and longing in that environment, so I only drank ginger and date tea or boiled water like everyone, and finally implemented the first experience of four days of fasting.

During the period, many students had vomiting, diarrhea and other HC, while I basically passed through smoothly, except for the first two days of some hunger and panic. However, the urination situation was special, every time the urine was light pink as watermelon juice in the few days of the fasting. I asked the coach about the reason of my condition. The answer was: kidney toxicity. Because I had taken Chinese and Western medicines for many years before, toxins had been deposited in my liver and kidneys, which detoxified through the fasting.

After having a fasting experience, in May, I encouraged my daughter to join me in the fasting, due to insufficient preparation in advance and my daughter's hunger, fasting was forced to stop in two days, which was considered an unsuccessful valley opening experience. Later, I realized that if you want to open fasting, you must first be fully mentally prepared, psychologically yearning, firm in action, set a goal and then not be disturbed by the outside world, so that it is easier to achieve fasting.

At the first time, I read the fasting record of the nine days of Riyue teacher on the forum, I started to feel the itch again. Thus, I made up my mind to implement the third fasting plan, and I finally passed the six-day fasting with ease.

In September, I read the nine-day sharing record of Teacher Riyue on the forum. I would like to try it again, so I made up my mind to implement the third fasting plan, so that I could easily spend the six days of fasting, finally.

There is my record for reference: On October 7, the first day of fasting, I was not uncomfortable. On October 8, the second day of fasting, I did Zen jogging for 30 minutes, Paida for an hour, and two times of Lajin for 30 minutes each time. I only drank ginger and date tea, without bowel movements and strong hunger, in a good spirit, and I worked as usual. On October 9, the third day of fasting, 1:30 am, I felt a slight pain in the liver area, promptly with the heart method silently to my body for a little hunger and dizziness. Thus, I drank a glass of plain water and felt better immediately; did 200 strokes of twisting, 5 minutes of Lajin, 15x2 each time in the morning and the evening in the lying position, and 30 minutes of Zen jogging. I did not poop 3 days, and went to work as usual.

October 10, the fourth day of the fasting, I did Zen jogging for half an hour, Lajin once in the morning and the evening, 15 min x 2 each time, and Paida for 1 hour. I only drank ginger and date tea, without discomfort and bowel movement, I worked normally. On October 11, the fifth day of the fasting, I did Zen jogging for 30 minutes, Paida for 1 hour, Lajin 15 min x 2. I felt a little weak when I woke up in the morning, drank some plain water and drank ginger and date tea, I was getting good, had the sense of hunger at afternoon, I felt good now and worked normally. I did not poop for five days. I would hope to have a carefree bowel movement and get rid of all the toxins. Fighting, my goal is six days. On October 12, the sixth day of the fasting, the scheduled plan was successfully completed, without being starved to death, I was still well, successful achieved the weight loss of one pound everyday. Please applaud me for encouragement.

## Change

One year ago, I took the plunge to stop taking all my medication, including the thyroid hormone drug Eugenol, which my doctor had told me that shall not stop taking medication without permission (I had been taking this drug for nine years), as my doctor had warned that patient with Hashimoto's thyroid disease is required lifelong medication and I should not stop taking medication without permission. Otherwise, I would be in danger of cardiac arrest. If you want to fight for your life, you must make the choice to overcome yourself and break the rules. Although there are few cases of Hashimoto's thyroiditis healed on the official website of PL, I believed that all illnesses are compound illnesses. All illnesses occur when the meridians are blocking, while all illnesses disappear when the meridians are unblocking.

In April this year, we had a physical examination in our unit. Although my thyroid indicators are not completely normal, the values are now better than when I was taking medication, which increased my confidence and motivation to continue PL. Yugong can move mountains with small progress everyday, I can see the hope of healing. My hypertension symptoms disappeared naturally after I stopped taking Eugenol, and my blood pressure now remains normal at 120/80. It seemed that the side effects of western medicine shall really not to be underestimated. My blood sugar, which was high in the past, has been largely controlled by PL. I can eat the occasional sweet treat that I can not to eat before. My close friends said that my body shape was slimmer than before, my complexion was better than before. My height had been increased by two centimeters through Lajin. I had recovered well from the scapulohumeral periarthritis, constipation, sleep and other conditions.

Certainly, PL is not a panacea for complex pathologies, it is not an accomplish in an action, especially for chronic diseases. If you want to be healthy, then PL must be a tug of war and a protracted battle. If we expect to get rid of all the diseases in the short term of PL, it is impossible. At present, I basically did Paida for one hour every day and Lajin for 20 to 30 minutes on each leg, lifted my leg with 4 Kg sandbags pressed, pulled down legs with 6 Kg sandbags pressed, combined with occasional Zen jogging, wall banging, waist twisting, foot soaking and others. All exercises are important to persevere. If PL is deemed as eating and sleeping, we would accept and love it, so that it becomes a habit of life, then I believe that health is not far from us.

I remembered that during the workshop, Mr. Xiao kept repeatedly emphasized this sentence: the Daoli should be separated, Dao refers to take action, Li refers to say, the key to PL is the word "action", action is the execution. There are many people around me who know that PL is a better way to improve self-healing. However, it is difficult to persist in it. Because they are afraid of the pain or they do not have the spare time, or they have convinced themselves without willing of change for themselves, including my family.

It is true that if I had not felt the pain or had not got the serious disease, I probably would have given up. However, when you find yourself with only one last straw in your life, you have to give it a shot. At least, it was a rewarding journey without costing anything.

Regarding PL, I have done a lot of communication and promotion work in the past year. I made 50 copies of the booklet *PL Self-Healing Manual* and distributed them to my relatives and friends. Meanwhile, the four discs purchased from the workshop were consolidated into one disc and burned 100 copies for distribution to friends who required them. I have held many simple PL gatherings for neighbors, relatives, classmates, friends and colleagues, and have participated in more than ten gatherings of PL held by the Shanghai group and acted as a partner training. All those around me with PL experiences had solved their own specific problems, I would not give any examples here.

### Concerns

First, I started involved with PL on a TV show when it was being promoted as a form of health. However, it took less than a year from my contact with PL due to the criticism of Mr. Xiao among the media.

As a medium channel for disseminating information, why are there two different voices in a short period of time? When dose media television be a medium for disseminating information? How can the people tell right from wrong in the dark? Where has the credibility of media gone when no investigation has been conducted and no right to speak has been taken out of context and had perpetrated a fraud?

Any citizen with a conscience knows the truth: the facts can be spoken out for themselves, and practice is the only test of truth. There are many people who have benefited from and are committed to PL. There are many brave people as Mr. Xiao Hongci, who had inherited and promoted PL. However, I have no idea how far PL can go. In the face of various pressures, PL method of self-healing can only blossom inside the walls at the stage. Fortunately, I can see that there are still many people who are actively promoting and practising PL self-healing method.

**Gratitude**

The changes in my body and mind over the past year of PL have been a source of great emotion for someone who had been through the ordeal of illness and pain. I am grateful to my parents for their nurturing love, my body, hair and skin stem from my parents. I was not able to cherish them properly, and I am ashamed. Those who love others shall love themselves first. Cherishing their own lives is the best reward for their parents. I am grateful to you for Paida with my uncontrollable crying when you did Paida me for many times, your shoulder is the most powerful thing that I can rely on; I am grateful to my daughter for being as sweet and warm as a small cotton jacket, having a pair of gentle hands to support me when I got sick and weak; I am grateful to the PL for giving me hope and a new life; I am grateful to the Shanghai PL communication group, Mr. Riyue, Mr. Xiao Mao and Mr. Sandstorm for your selfless dedication and love. I am grateful to our fellows, I can feel warm and proud of the group; thanks, Xiangcao, 21 g, Qingfeng Mingyue, Lianhua Yijiu, Stone, Qingqingcao, Mr. Tang and so on, who I have never met before. Thanks for your trust and encouragement, you have given me enough confidence and courage, let's work together and cheer for health! Cheers for our life!

I would like to commemorate my first anniversary of PL with this article. I could hope that those who have had similar experiences as me, or those fellows who are still confused, and wandering on the road of seeking medical treatment, they can learn from it and take less detour or wrong paths, join PL exchange group and witness miracles with their actions. I oversee my health. Once Paida will benefit the whole family for entire life, the whole family can also benefit from Paida.

--Jinghua Shuiyue, December 18, 2012

As the author of the previous case, the author's illnesses increased with the medication used, she had the physical examination in 2003 that revealed thyroiditis, myometritis and endometriosis simultaneously. The treatment included taking medication and conducting an operation to remove an ovarian cyst. The breast enlargement, fibroids, hyperlipidemia, hypertension and diabetes were developed one after another in 2008. How could a normal person have so many illnesses in a short period of time if the large number of medications taken that did not have a negative effects? Therefore, she lamented, "When will I stop taking these pills? I even feel that death is not far away, and I am helpless in the face of my own body."

Illness is a decision that the mind uses the body for some purpose. It is still the mind's decision to become sicker. The aggravation of the disease and the increased types of diseases are still decisions of the mind. It means that sickness comes from the mind. Because only the mind can make decisions. After PL for one year, she summed up the cause of her illness as below: "I was tired of running around, focused on gains and losses, loved to save face, loved to show off, loved to lose my temper. In short, I wanted too much and gave up too little. The imbalance in my mind creates an imbalance in my body..." It is all the state of the heart, and the state of the mind determines the state of body. However, we are in the same state. People can realize that the mind can be changed and discover that PL can help people to improve the mind in particular, which is a huge step forward. Throughout the self-healing process, it is the process of changing the mentality.

For example, a two-hour session of moxibustion in 2010 healed her of menstrual cramps that had been a pain in the neck for years. "This experience completely overturned my views on the so-called formal hospitals and expert professors." The function of moxibustion is the same as PL, for opening up the meridians. One year later. When she discovered PL method, she read the book "three times. After reading the booklet I exclaimed, "That's great! It was so good! ...There is no place to step on iron shoes, and it takes no effort to get it." How many people have the excitement of her learning PL for the first time? It can only be said that the torture of being sick, the experience of moxibustion and medicine had finally prepared her mind to accept PL, which the true mind of experiencer.

However, the confidence in PL shall be built by experiences and it can not be achieved overnight. After a month of Paida on the universal area, she noticed that her sleep had improved, and her heart was not panicking. The improvement in her symptoms boosted her confidence of Paida. However, she did not know until then that her worst illness was heart disease, while sleep, panic attacks, even hypertension and thyroid disease were just complications of heart disease. Apart from heart disease, the deeper illness was actually heart disease: doubt and fear. "Are the articles on Mr. Xiao's blog true or not? Are the results really amazing?" It was her mindset before she joined the camp.

However, once she attended the camp, the healing effects saw were beyond her imagination. While the physical healing effects of PL are no longer surprising. Because there is obvious effectiveness to everyone, the more profound and hidden healing effects are the resolution of deep-seated mental illnesses. The negative emotions and misconceptions are significantly improved by the collective patting and sharing of the heart. In particular, the sharing and resonance of the mind can create a huge energy field that is unimaginable when did Lajin alone. Because when many peoples work together towards a common goal, the combined power is far greater than the sum of the individuals. Importantly, it can penetrate deep into the blockages of the mind and dissolves heart disease. Thus, she wrote, "The camp not only taught me PL techniques and mental cultivation methods, but also taught me an optimistic attitude towards life. Many participants were in tears at the sharing session before we left. I suddenly felt a sense of rebirth at the moment when I left the camp." It was clearly spiritual uplifting.

The article is her reflections on the first anniversary of Paida. It seemed from the article that she stopped all medication when she first started PL, a seemingly excessive act that is clearly the result of heartache and pain. At least, the mind has experienced the clinical results of taking medication and increasing medication, which is the continuous deterioration of the condition and the increase of heart disease. Thus, "One year ago I took the plunge and stopped all medication, including the thyroid hormone drug - Eugenol, which my doctor had told me that shall not stop taking medication without permission (I had been taking this drug for nine years), as my doctor had warned that patient with Hashimoto's thyroid disease is required lifelong medication and I should not stop taking medication without permission. Otherwise, I would be in danger of cardiac arrest."

However, "We had a check-up at my unit in April this year (i.e. four months after PL and stopping the medication). Although my thyroid indicators were not completely normal, the values were getting now better without the medication, compared with taking medication, which has increased my confidence and motivation to continue PL." More clinically valuable results shall come in the future, "My hypertension symptoms disappeared naturally after I stopped taking Eugenol. At present, my blood pressure has remained normal at 120/80. It seemed that the side effects of western medicine should not be underestimated!" Compare to the previous doctor's advice that stopping the drug would cause heart danger, her hypertension even became normal after stopping the drug. Hypertension is just a symptom of heart disease, which could indicate that taking this drug is only dangerous to the heart. If you take drugs for a long time, you will damage your heart in the long term, so your blood pressure will be high for a long time. You will have to stop taking anti-hypertensive drugs to generate more negative effects.

In addition, the result of stopping the medication and adding PL is that high blood sugar, scapulohumeral periarthritis, constipation and sleep and other conditions recovered well. These symptoms are characterized by blockage of the heart, pericardium, large intestine, lung, liver and small intestine meridian, which are also responsible for the formation of conditions, such as thyroid disease and hypertension. It can be seen that although the symptoms and names of the diseases are diverse, they are all different bodily reactions to the same blockage of the meridian network. In other words, although there are various forms with the same connotation, which are caused by the blocked meridians. Anxiety and heart disease are her main diseases. All symptoms are merely complications of heart disease.

Once the simple truth is understood, healing can be much easier. However, the problem is the difficulty and complexity of the human heart, rather than the difficulty of treating these illnesses and the complexity of the methods. It seemed from the author's reflections on one year of Paida that what she really changed was her own mind. In particular, the knowledge that came from her mind: her knowledge about the causes of illness and healing, medical treatment and medicine was completely changed. She wrote this article when there was a great deal of criticism of PL in the media, and the critics of PL had one common: they had never used PL in clinical trials, nor had they ever researched people who had experimented with PL or attended PL camps. Why do they hate this simple method that can give people relief from pain?

The answer is obvious: because their knowledge and insights. Based on the knowledge and the perception in their minds, the good heal and simple method without drugs is impossible. Even the approval or rejection of a treatment by modern medicine requires a basic prerequisite: a clinical trial. The problem is that these people do not even think about experimenting. For the extent to which PL is so effective and simple that is far beyond their vision, knowledge and even imagination. How can a complex, misshapen mind possibly appreciates the simplicity of the principle?

## 1-15 Effect of PL on hyperthyroidism, post-stroke

Linda Preliana, 49 years old, living in Bandung, Indonesia.

I had been suffering from hyperthyroidism since 2010. On April 30, 2012, I had my first radioactive treatment. Because the results were still not satisfactory, I had another radioactive treatment on the September 6 of the same year.

After treatment by a number of professors and endocrine specialists, my eyes and heart were highly allergic to all medications. Because of the hyperthyroidism, I had a rapid heartbeat, a high and weak pulse even when I was not fatigued. Besides, I started to tremble. I was easily agitated, sad and emotional.

In 2013, my eyes started to swell and bulge out and eventually became double vision, so that I was banned from driving by my doctor. I started to become desperate and could not do anything, not even watch TV as I could only see it with one eye.

I was also sad that my skin was allergic to the sunray and when the temperature got hot, my skin became itched and left scratch marks everywhere. There were dark rash spots all over my face for too many hormones.

Annoyingly, I could not take any medication, even though they are right there on the shelf. To reduce the stress on my eye nerves, my eye doctor had prescribed high doses of steroids. A more obvious side effect was that my face swelled up into a round face and gained weight.

One night after taking the medication, my tongue swelled, my ear cavity and entire body itched, and I went to the emergency room at 2:00 am. Because I had trouble breathing. Before the blisters showed up, my skin was itchy everyday. It happened repeatedly every time I took the medication. Since then, I must resort to non-medical treatments, including acupuncture, hitting vital points and massage.

On December 10, 2013, Ms. Nensi introduced me to the couple Hanafi, who had come to Bandung, Indonesia to promote PL. I did PL at GOR, their event venue in Bandung, and did Paida at home a few times without seriousness. I did not know if PL has a sustained improvement in test results. I only knew that after Mr Hanafi came to GOR, I did PL once a day lasting for 14 days and my free thyroxine test results improved. The thyroid stimulating hormone had not changed in three years, also started to change. However, I still did not PL regularly and had to be urged by Ms. Nensi to do it. There was some effectiveness. However, it is still a bit undulate and unstable.

When I attended PL seminar and the subsequent workshop in Bandung at the end of June 2015, I worked more diligently on PL and I noticed that my knees did not hurt or rattle when I went up and down the stairs.

In the morning, I woke up with more refreshed feelings. The test results suggest improvement of indicators. The cholesterol and other indicators are normalized. The most recent indicator comparison was on August 18, 2015. The endocrinologist at Boromeus Hospital asked me what was going on with PL and she wanted to see it on Youtube, she also asked me to write it down on paper. She asked me several times what was going on about my bruises frequently (was she thought it as the domestic violence??). From the doctor's feedback, PL had been improving my body well and I should continue to PL.

My 81 year-old mother had a stroke in 2010. She was laying in bed for one year and could not take care of herself. For two years received acupuncture twice a week, then once a week. She also received electrotherapy once. Eventually, she was able to sit up with difficulties, she was difficult to walk, with the limited movement of her right arm and she was unable to speak fluently, it was the living condition of my mother before the Muslim New Year on July 17, 2015.sS

Seeing the improvement in my health, some people around me, including my mother, started PL on her knees and hands in the morning and evening. A lot of purple and black bruises came out around the knees and hands, while the bruises quickly receded. She felt cold shivers that night and the next morning, she was able to move her right thumb and little finger.

This morning, my mother was so happy that she showed me that she had the strength in her right arm to pat her right knee. Thank God for that. There is nothing else wrong with her and I would hope that she will soon be able to walk normally again.

———Linda Preliana, 20-08-2015

Unlike these previous cases, the author of this article was forced to stop taking the medication voluntarily. "Annoyingly, I could not take any medications, even though they are right there on the shelf." It is the result of having had two radioactive treatments up front. "After treatment by a number of professors and endocrine specialists, my eyes and heart were highly allergic to all medications. Because of the hyperthyroidism, I had a rapid heartbeat, and a high and weak pulse even when I was not fatigued. Besides, I started to tremble. I was easily agitated, sad and emotional." The iodine 131 mentioned in the previous case is a radioactive drug.

From the view of the symptoms, it seemed that the heart, lung, pericardium and liver meridians are blocking. In fact, it is obvious heart disease and depression. While two diseases are not easily diagnosed, the indicators of other diseases are easily checked. All of the treatments revolve around the obvious symptoms and indicators. "To reduce the stress on my eye nerves, my eye doctor had prescribed high doses of steroids. A more obvious side effect was that my face swelled up into a round face and gained weight. At one night, after taking the medication, my tongue swelled, my ear cavity and entire body itched, and I went to the emergency room at 2:00 am. Because I had trouble breathing. Before the blisters showed up, my skin was itchy everyday. It happened repeatedly every time when I took the medication. Since then, I have had to resort to non-medical treatments, including acupuncture, hitting vital points and massage."

It is the reason that she came to receive PL, she really had no alternative method. The couple Hanafis returned to their homeland of Indonesia to promote PL after attending an experiential camp in Australia where they had extraordinary healing results. "I PL once a day and did it again after 14 days, my test results of free thyroxine and thyroid stimulating hormone was changed and improved, which had not changed for three years passed. However, I still do not PL regularly and have to be urged by Ms. Nensi to do it." It was the initial clinical result, the initiative and intensity of PL could not be compared to the previous cases. Thus, the efficacy was limited to it.

In 2015, she attended my first workshop in Indonesia in Bandung. Her knee pain was healed. Moreover, "I woke up and felt more energized in the morning. The test results suggested improvement, including normal cholesterol and other indicators. From the doctor's feedback, my body has been improved so well by PL that I should continue PL". She had further boosted her confidence in PL by attending the camp. She also found that it was effective in improving the post-stroke sequelae by PL on her mother. How far she can implement PL only depends on her confidence. Because confidence determines her ability to act. The fact that she was forced to take PL. The situation that she could not take her medication shall be deemed as an opportunity, the opportunity of whether she will persist depends on her heart.

## 1-16 Hyperthyroidism, Amenorrhoea, Constipation, Depression and Severe Weakness

It is Ms. Qiu. I am living in Massachusetts, USA. I have been practicing and benefiting from PL method since 2009 when I learned about it from the Sina Blog of Mr. Xiao.

In 2009. When I was 33 years old, I experienced a series of serious illnesses including hyperthyroidism, amenorrhoea, severe constipation and extraordinary weakness. Firstly, I lost 40 pounds in one year for hyperthyroidism (from 119 pounds to 79 pounds); secondly, I did not get my period for several months, or precisely speaking, only 1-2 periods a year since 2007; thirdly, I was extremely difficult to have a bowel movement, even though I really felt like I need the bowel movement for only 1-2 times a week; finally, it was the most troubling that my physical energy was so low and I could not manage the normal meals or shopping. Finally, it was the most troubling that I have a low level of fitness that I am unable to carry out shopping, cooking and other normal daily tasks. Therefore, I can be unable to look after myself and my three-year-old child. These health problems interfere with me negatively that I often feel it is worse than death to live in the condition. As a natural consequence, my temper got worse, and I became more depressed.

I saw the various doctors and specialists in the mainstream medicine, while the hormonal treatments were suitable to me. I turned to traditional Chinese medicine and other natural remedies, such as moxibustion, acupuncture, aromatherapy and so on. These non-mainstream methods have helped me a lot and have improved my health. However, I shall find an effective, independent, inexpensive and convenient method. Therefore, when I came across PL method on Mr. Xiao's blog, I immediately felt that my prayers had been answered.

I started practising PL diligently at home everyday and never paid Mr. Xiao a penny. Gradually, my weight returned to my best weight (100-105 pounds), my periods returned to normal, my daily bowel movements were normal, and my energy needs for daily living returned to normal. More importantly, my attitude about life became more positive and in the spring of 2014, after attending a workshop organized by Mr. Xiao in California, I became pregnant in winter, 2014. I gave birth to another beautiful, healthy baby in the autumn of 2015. During my pregnancy and postpartum period, I experienced many difficulties physically and emotionally. PL always helped me through difficulties and made me stronger and healthier. At present, I am 42 years old with two children. I feel healthier and more energetic than I did nine years ago. My family and friends have witnessed my transformation and have come to accept PL. I have solved their various problems by PL, such as colds, stomach aches, coughs, muscle strains, dizziness, headaches, shoulder pains and so on.

Apart from greatly improving my health, PL has also triggered a change in my thinking, so that I believe that everyone can be their own doctor, reconnecting with their own body, taking charge of themselves, and regaining their own awareness and perception of every moment of their lives. Because of my personal experience, I have nothing but endless gratitude to Mr. Xiao and PL. I have a deep respect for mainstream and non-mainstream therapies and for doctors and healers. I also strongly believe that people should have the right to choose the Therapy that best suits them and take any possible risks and consequences that may result from it. May more people can learn about PL and turn themselves into their own healers, to heal their bodies, minds and spirits.

-- Ms. Qiu, July 9, 2018

It is another classic case of a heart condition evolving into a heart disease that is not easily diagnosed. Then a series of complications arise from it. When a person suffers from hyperthyroidism, it means that the heart, pericardium, lung, large intestine, small intestine and Tri-jiao meridians are all blocked, with the central and Pericardium meridians being the most severely blocked. Because the onset location is in the neck where these meridians pass. What is the cause? It can only be the heart, the invisible mind, where you can feel negative emotions and conflicted thoughts and dissatisfaction, while it is difficult to find biomarkers until hyperthyroidism appears. However, as the lesion is in the neck, it is difficult to associate it with any connection to the blockage of the heart meridian. Moreover, Western medicine does not have the concept of meridians.

It was only after reading this report many times that I noticed a detail: although her various illnesses worsened in 2009, her amenorrhoea began in 2007. The child was only one year old at the time, who had obviously already experienced a number of illnesses after giving birth. As for her amenorrhea, it was unlikely that she did not visit hospital, doctor must have given her hormonal medication. Perhaps two years of medication led to her further illnesses. Three conditions: hyperthyroidism, amenorrhoea and constipation, all of them can be interpreted in Western medical theory as inflammation caused by the overactive microglia. Why was there weakness in the body? It is the "Leaky Gut" caused by the inflammation of the intestines, so that it was difficult to remove toxins and prevent the absorption of nutrients, people could be weaker. In the book *Complete Recovery written by* Dr. Kaplan, there are several cases where this has led to a range of symptoms such as weakness, pain and depression. If one went to a gynaecologist or internist for amenorrhoea, can you imagine what else they would do besides hormones and antibiotics? She has tried all methods, so that she refused to do the clinical trial again. She got rid of all the diseases by PL once, rather than just treating amenorrhea. Because the diseases may be complicated. However, it was just a bunch of blocked meridians. You can be healed by opening them up! It is just so simple!

Each person can only deal with the stress by his or her own knowledge and insight, that is, the individual ideas has acquired through a lifetime of education. She could figure out the stress faced only by herself, while her physical illness was an objective indication of the result of unresolved internal stress. Menorrhagia, hyperthyroidism and constipation are thereby caused. Anxiety and heart disease are difficult to diagnose, they are a major source of disease. However, diseases can be diagnosed by Paida. Because their common feature is a failure of the heart and pericardium meridians. She did not know so many theoretical details, just follow the basic method that she learned from the Internet. If you pat on the universal areas, the first three meridians are the heart, pericardium and lung meridians, all the meridians of the body can be unblocked by Lajin.

The author's strength can be concluded as the good perception and strong execution. Since she already had a desire in her heart for simple and effective natural remedies, the knowledge was already moving in the right direction, so she found that PL can heal her diseases. Is that the heart healing? The intensity of her daily PL will naturally achieve to resolve all diseases. Many people who have experienced the benefits of self-patting at home, she has improved her technique and mindfulness since attending the camp. Her summary also highlights another shift above the physical improvements, a change in her mind. She has realized that the doctor of human being is the own mind. Paida can help you to be aware of your mind and focus on the present moment. The elevation of the mind is subtle and you can realize it in the clinic and your life, and the change is the real purpose of the body being sick.

## 1-17 Severe hyperthyroidism, amenorrhea, depression and other 11 diseases healed by Paida

I am 31 years old, who had many physical health problems before PL.

1. Six years of hyperthyroidism: Protruding eyes, shaky hands, and thick neck.
2. Irregular periods: Frequent amenorrhea for 6 months and there was black blood in the occasional periods.
3. Depression: I was irritable, easily agitated and cry, had a negative outlook on life, and wanted to commit suicide.
4. From a young age, no matter whether I have a cold or get inflamed, the tonsils could swell up and eventually ulcerate.
5. The waist could be stiff for a little bit of housework, and it was uncomfortable like a plank of wood.
6. I had been in the state of cold all year round, and the various anti-inflammatory drugs shall be prepared at home all year round.
7. Inexplicable dry cough, dry cough for no reason.
8. Loose stools.
9. Since hyperthyroidism is serious, I could not get pregnant, which is troublesome.
10. I could not stand washing and mopping the floor for the sciatica in my right buttock.
11. Liver function was not normal for long term use of western medicine.

All conditions above are my status and symptoms before PL. I was born in 1987 with hyperthyroidism for 6 years. When I was 23 years old, I was diagnosed with hyperthyroidism after her neck swelled up overnight for anger and getting inflamed. Since then, I had been on a vicious cycle of medication and blood draws. After taking the medicine for several years, not only did it not get better, but it became more serious. I had drunk a lot of Chinese medicine medicament. The results were not ideal. I have eaten various health care products, eaten for more than a year, the money has not been spent, and various adverse reactions have come out before stopping.

It was painful to have this disease for 6 years, and people were desperate and helpless. In April 2015, I found PL method promoted by Mr. Xiao Hongci on the Internet. I learned that the disease was caused by the lack of meridians, and I immediately put it into action! From the first day of Paida, I did not tell my family, secretly stopped all the medicine, there were great side effects of hyperthyroidism western medicine. Thus, I decisively stopped the drug by myself. I read the cases written by the teacher's blog everyday and the *PL Self-healing Method Manual* to study. I persisted with Paida more than 3 hours everyday. At first, each leg could only be stretched for 3 minutes. And it becomes more than 20 minutes per leg. During the period, I met HC: I was so flustered in the middle of the night that I could not breathe, and finally slapped the inside of my arm to solve it. In August 2015, I found out that I was pregnant, and the hospital checked all the indicators normally, and my liver function returned to normal.

Problems were improved by PL:

1. Hyperthyroidism was healed, hands did not shake at all, my neck became slim and normal, eyes were also gradually recovered.
2. Periods were normal in red, rather than black blood as before. Periods were on time until I was pregnancy.
3. I was not depressed anymore, I love to laugh, I found that there are many good people, I no longer argued with my

husband for no reason, and my family found that I became better tempered.
4. The body immunity was improved, the occasionally cold was healed by Paida and drinking ginger date soup. I had not taken any medicine after Paida.
5. The problem of back pain was 90% solved, which is no pain without over-strain.
6. Tonsils did not swell and ulcerate.
7. The stool was formed.
8. I had pregnant and delivered smoothly, the baby was healthy, who is two weeks old now.
9. Liver function was normal.
10. The sciatica in my buttocks was healed by Lajin once.
11. Basically, I have a few flatus vocis every morning, and I can discharge the turbid gas.

There are all real changes in my body. I am so lucky to come into contact with PL when I was desperate, so that I was no longer helpless, and my life trajectory had been transformed!

I love Mr. Xiao! I love the people who have helped me! I love PL! I have also been quietly promoting PL for the past few years, with family, online friends, netizens, and neighbours, and I had helped many people. PL is a voluntary action. I also tell people to read PL notes in advance, understand HC process, learn, and practice, without doing it blindly.

Thank you again, Mr. Xiao! A valuable person in my life! Without you, I would not have my healthy child and the colourful life now.

-- Ms. Hao, August 12, 2018

Hyperthyroidism, amenorrhea and depression in this case was similar to the previous case, except that the intestinal inflammation was in the opposite direction, with loose stools in this case and constipation in the previous case. According to Western medicine's theory of microglia and leaky gut, there was obvious leaky gut syndrome, with all 11 conditions being the result of inflammation caused by microglia. However, as in the above example, the author was unaware that her worst illness was heart disease. Many conditions are complications of heart disease in fact.

In terms of gynecological diseases, the previous case was only 1-2 periods per year, this case was "frequent amenorrhoea for six months, with the occasional periods in black." In addition, she "was unable to get pregnant for severe hyperthyroidism became a big problem." Her depression was even worse, "with a negative outlook on life and a desire to commit suicide." If the heart-made disease is not well understood, this case is illustrated with personal clinical experience, "When I was 23 years old, I was diagnosed with hyperthyroidism after her neck swelled up overnight for anger and getting inflamed." Inflammation is a heart disease caused by blockage of heart meridian and pericardium meridian. There is no doubt about heart disease, you can show the degree of blockage of the heart meridian and pericardium meridian if you pat inside the elbow on the spot. Because the heart is the ruler of the sovereign, the king's fault is often taken by the ministers. Thus, the symptoms of heart disease are then manifested by the swelling of neck. However, if one analyses the meridians, one can clearly see that the enlargement is at the place where the heart and pericardium meridians, the large and small intestine meridians pass through. There is also a problem with the stool. The intestines and stomach are damaged, the mechanism of detoxification and absorption of nutrients is completely chaotic. The microglia theory is interpreted that the cranial nerves and intestinal nerves are inflamed. The solution for Western medicine is the use of various medicines.

The above example mentions that the author could not accept the use of hormones to treat hyperthyroidism in Western medicine. In this case, she used such drugs for six years, and as a result, "Since then, I have been on a vicious cycle of medication and blood draws. After taking the medicine for several years, not only did it not get better, but it became more and more serious." As a result, "From the first day of Paida, I did not tell my family, secretly stopped all the medicine, there were great side effects of hyperthyroidism western medicine. Thus, I decisively stopped the drug by myself." I certainly do not advocate stopping medication at random; we should analyse it specifically and consult a doctor. Her decision to stop her medication seems be clear, i.e. the result of a clinical trial. What should I do if I have more disease from taking medication for 6 years?

If you do not understand heart disease, the clear verification can be obtained from her HC, "I was so flustered in the middle of the night that I could not breathe. Finally, I did Paida the inside of my arm to heal it." This HC is a heart attack, which is also easily resolved by her patting on the heart and pericardium meridians. What an accurate diagnosis of HC and an effective self-healing! Each HC is not only a diagnosis, it is a self-healing. She started PL in April and became pregnant in August, which indicated that her gynecological problems had been resolved. She also wrote that "Periods were normal in red, rather than black blood as before. Periods were on time until I was pregnant." It means that in less than four months her gynecological problems had resolved. Of course, a total of 11 medical conditions had also been resolved, including a heart condition that she did not know about, and depression diagnosed, "I was not depressed anymore, I love to laugh, I found that there are many good people, I no longer argued with my husband for no reason, and my family found that I became have better temper." Faced with the same people and the world, her interpretation is different and her mood has been improved. It is the result of PL's self-healing to improve knowledge and insight.

It seems that PL is a natural way of healing the heart in the process of healing the body. When depression is dissolved, it means that the heart meridian and pericardium meridian is more unblocking and heart disease is dissolved. It means that the heart meridian and the pericardium meridian will be more unblocking, and heart disease will certainly be resolved. Hyperthyroidism, amenorrhoea, constipation and loose stools and other diseases resulting complications will also naturally be resolved. In fact, PL is not used for a specific disease. However, the disordered energy field that can cause the disease indicates the blocked meridians. The main cause of the blockage is the invisible mind. If the mind is still unhappy after the illness, or the mind is depressed again for some reason at any time, it means that people's perception is not improved. They do not put down the obstacles in their hearts, they are too serious about the world, it is normal to get sick again or the old disease recurs or intensifies. Because the cause stems from the heart, it has been not resolved yet.

## 1-18 Eight diseases of patient with hyperthyroidism healed by PL

My name is Xiao Xu. I found Guangzhou lactation consultant Ms. Yu through my cousin. My cousin had mastitis during breastfeeding and her fever reached 40 degrees. After the hospital failed to heal her fever, she found a Guangzhou lactation therapist, Ms. Yu, who healed her by Paida. At this time, my cousin had appendicitis with severe pain, so she went to hospital for emergency treatment and the doctor asked her to be hospitalized for an operation. My cousin refused and asked PL to heal her. I thought that Ms. Yu should be able to help me with my illness too.

In 2002, I had a strange illness: two tumor-like lumps protruded from my neck against my throat and veins protruded from under my eyelids. In 2005, I suddenly gained weight from 45 Kg to 64 Kg. In 2011, I started to lose weight again, I kept seeking medical help during this period. However, it did not help.

In 2002, I suffered from a strange illness: two tumor-like masses protruded from my neck against my throat, and the blue tendons under my eyelids protruded. After taking Paida once, the lump disappeared. However, the throat began to feel a little uncomfortable, I did not care. In 2005, the whole person suddenly became fat, from 45 Kg to 64 Kg. In 2011, I began to lose weight again, I constantly sought medical treatment and medicine during this period, while I was not healed.

After I delivered my child in 2013, my health was getting worsened:

1. Cold hands and feet, needing socks to sleep at night;
2. Insomnia;
3. Stools once every few days;
4. Bloated stomach and heavy breath;
5. No saliva in the mouth and uncomfortable dryness;
6. I cannot kneel on the ground with toes hurting:
7. Whole body was stiff;
8. No sweating after strenuous exercise
9. The expression on the face is getting stiff, I can not smile entire day, with no interest in anything, as a living dead person.

Recently, I have had a cold and cough for over a month, and I have been seeing doctors and taking medication in my hometown and never got better. My throat was getting more uncomfortable, I felt that there was something stuck in it and I could not cough it up, and my neck was hard to the touch. My family urged me to go to hospital for a check-up. However, I did not want to go for unnecessary tests. Because I knew that the hospital would not be able to heal me even if a bad disease is revealed by the tests. I told Ms. Yu about my condition, I would hope to get her help.

Ms. Yu told me to go back and read *PL Self-Healing Manual* and the cases of Mr. Xiao on his blog first. I should read and understand them before deciding. Thus, I went back and started to follow Mr. Xiao's blog and read PL *Self-Healing Manual*, and started to learn how to Paida on my own, while I could not really do it. After a month of consideration, I decided to receive PL treatment from Ms. Yu.

There were the changes in my PL regimen:

After the first day of PL, I had phlegm in my throat and could cough it out, which Ms. Yu said that it was a good sign.

On the second day, after I started Zen jogging, flat shaking, standing meditation and PL, I felt more comfortable in my throat and stopped coughing in the middle of the night. However, I did not have a bowel movement for 2 days, while I had the urge to have bowel movement. It would not come out. Ms. Yu told me to start PL on the third day. I was worried that I would not have anything to eat, and I would not have bowel movement. However, Ms. Yu told me that do not worry, it would be easier to pass stools and detoxify the body.

On the third day, I started to come back to life and continued with Zen jogging, flat shaking, standing meditation, PL moxibustion and drinking ginger and date tea. My stomach started to move and there were noises. Ms. Yu said that it was a prelude to bowel detoxification, sending signals. At night, I still can not have bowel movement and keep farting. While I expelled a lot of waste water and cold, cold Qi came out of my hands and feet during Paida, water came out of my palms, and a lot of cold water came out of my middle abdomen with moxibustion.

On the fourth day, I continued to fast, Zen jogging, flat shake, Standing meditation, stretch, Paida on my face and other parts of my body, moxibustion and drink ginger and date tea. At night, before I went to bed, I suddenly could not hold it anymore and had to go to the toilet. I wanted to defecate. As a result, I pulled out a lot of green loose stools, which were floating on the toilet with many bubbles. Ms. Yu said that it was turbid gas and feces in the stomach, and I feel so relaxed after Lajin.

On the fifth day, I defecated again early in the morning, I pulled out all the past poop that was as black as asphalt. After defecation, I felt very comfortable and relaxed entirely, my facial muscles were also alive, and I naturally showed a smile and a smile from the heart, I saw hope. Because of the weather, I didn't Zen jogging, and I did flat throwing and twisting exercises in the hall. After these exercises, I continued PL and drank ginger and date tea. I felt so hungry that I wanted to steal some food, while I persevered and kept on it. I was cleaning up the toxins from my body and starve these poisonous cells. When Ms. Yu helped me check, the muscles on my body were irregular particles by touching. Skin was loose and inelastic; Ms. Yu told me that the muscle skin of healthy people shall be smooth and elastic.

On the sixth day, I continued to fast, Zen jogging, flat shake and Standing meditation. Ms. Yu said that my Qi and blood started to come up. Because I used to be breathless and lazy to talk. At present, I love to talk and laugh. I also had uncomfortable reactions, such as panic, vomiting and hiccups during PL period. Ms. Yu had spoken to me beforehand and read examples on the blog of Mr. Xiao, I was not afraid to stick to PL in the face of HC.

On the seventh day, I had Zen jogging in the morning, Ms. Yu taught me to Lajin with big steps and Standing meditation. From that day, I was able to eat. I had millet congee in the morning and a small bowl of Tianqi soup at noon, while I did not eat any dinner. In the past two days, Ms. Yu basically helped me with the moxibustion treatment, which was comfortable. The whole process was painful and enjoyable. When I was bawling in pain, Ms. Yu released my mood and patiently guided me to realize that my diseases were caused by my bad attitude, bad emotions, and bad lifestyle habits.

After seven days of PL regimen, my body has changed a lot:

1. No coughing;
2. No pain in my toes on my bended knees;
3. My bowel movements are better;
4. The blue veins under my eyes have almost disappeared;
5. My neck is more flexible to rotate left and right back and forth;
6. The skin on the whole face is smoother and more elastic after Paida.
7. I feel more confident, and I can smile naturally now, as I could not smile before.
8. My hands and feet are warmer at night and I feel relaxed, so I feel lighter without drugs. Thank you!

I am grateful to Ms. Yu and Ms. Zhou Xia for bringing me into contact with PL. I am also grateful to Mr. Xiao for his selfless dedication in spreading PL Self-Healing Method! From now on, I will take good care of my body, adhere to PL, and spread the health concept of PL Self-Healing Method to the people around me!

--Xiao Xu, 2015.1.16

The most significant characteristic of author in this case is her instinctive avoidance of hospitals. She listed nine symptoms, which were all related to thyroid disease. She had a cold and cough for over a month, "I felt something stuck in my throat, I could not cough it up, and my neck felt hard to the touch. My family urged me to visit hospital for a check-up. However, I did not want to go for unnecessary tests. I knew the hospital would not be able to heal me if the tests were bad."

This instinctive resistance to hospitals was clearly related to the surgery and medication she was received and given after being diagnosed with hyperthyroidism. She said, "I did not have surgery, I was treated conservatively. I took the liquid medicine once, and the lump disappeared, my throat started to feel a bit uncomfortable." It is probably the reason why the throat problem has continued to the current. What medicine could be taken to make the lump disappear immediately? We can only guess that it was some kind of hormonal or radioactive drug. Certainly, "In 2005, the whole person suddenly became fat, from 45 Kg to 64 Kg. In 2011, I began to lose weight again, I constantly sought medical treatment and medicine during this period, while I was not healed" Apart from the negative effects of medication, there is no ordinary food that can achieve sudden loss and gain of weight for one person, is it right? Perhaps, it is a memory of her fear of hospital medication.

From her list of symptoms, the inoperative meridians can be observed. Insomnia is a blockage in the heart and pericardium meridians, which are also common to anxiety and heart disease; constipation and bloating are blockages in the large intestine and stomach meridians; lack of sweating and coughing are blockages in the lung meridians. Blockage of the heart, pericardium, lung, large intestine and stomach meridians is the main cause of thyroid disease. In short, the area from the neck to the collarbone is where the six meridians (three Yang and three Yin meridians) of the hand follow, where the thyroid gland is located. Look at the other symptoms: no saliva in the mouth, cold hands and feet, and stiffness of the entire body and facial expressions are complications of thyroid disease.

It was known that the relevant meridians are not are not connected, it is easy to understand the clinical practice of PL. On the first day, the inner side of the arm was patted usually, where the heart, lung and pericardium meridians were located, there was phlegm in the throat that can cough out immediately. It is actually the heart and lung meridian to open up the Qi to produce two types of HC: (1) Dissolve the foci for phlegm; (2) Expel the phlegm, which requires Qi to dissolve and rush out, so it is called as HC. In the middle night of the second day, I was not cough again. At the third day to the sixth day, fasting, PL, moxibustion, Standing meditation and other methods were still insisted. There were many HC: Emission of exhaust gas and cold Qi, coldness of hands and feet, and water was expelled, cold water gas came out from Zhongguan acupoint (abdomen) by moxibustion. On the fourth and fifth days, although she did not eat, she excreted the stools: green loose stools, with bubbles floating, which were obviously a great cleansing of many kinds of old toxins. On the sixth day, she became hot and sweaty. Previously, she did not sweat even when doing strenuous exercise. It is a symptom of HC that opens the heart and lung meridians, as the heart can change the fluid into sweat, while the lungs are the mainstay of the skin. The blockage of the heart and lung meridians is the main cause of thyroid disease.

HC that made her cry is the deepest HC, which dissolves and expels the heart toxins, i.e. all kinds of repressed negative emotions. It is the main cause of all illnesses, such as heart disease and hyperthyroidism. Therefore, the author, under PL and enlightenment of Ms. Yu, "realized that her diseases were caused by her bad mind, bad emotions and bad habits of life." In short, diseases can be all created by heart, and the mentality, emotions, and the habits can be all controlled by the mind.

The eight symptoms listed plus the fever and sweating are nine symptoms in total. In fact, the most important improvement is the $7^{th}$ symptom: "I feel more confident, I used to be unable to smile, now I can smile naturally." It is not only an improvement in the symptoms of hyperthyroidism, but also a revival of the mind.

## 1-19 Hyperthyroidism, post-surgery symptoms, tumor indicators improved by Paida

Ms. Liu Ying and Paida fellows:

Good evening, everyone. I would like to share with you my bonding and harvesting of PL.

I saw PL on the Internet in 2009. Because I love and believe in Chinese medicine. At that time, I took it home randomly and did not know how to learn it. Thus, I stopped PL because I felt it had no effect.

Later, in 2015 and 2016, my physical examination found that some tumor indicators were not good (4 tumors), and I had been in a sub-healthy state, I was afraid. Suddenly, I remembered PL, I felt that it could help me, so I checked on the Internet and signed up for the latest 7-day training camp in Xi'an.

That 7-day camp was still fresh in my mind and turned many of my idea's upside down. First, I learned about PL systematically, tried fasting for the first time (at that time, I was internally repulsed, so I only did fast for two days). When I went to the camp and saw the condition of the instructors and my friends, I was convinced of my faith in PL.

After 7-days training and roughly 6 months of Paida at home, I went for a review, which indicated that 2 of 4 indicators had improved and other 2 indicator had dropped a lot, without taking any medication. PL was real and effective. However, that is the bad character of people. When the condition becomes better, people start to become lazy. In the following years, I occasionally conducted Paida and really did not do enough.

At the end of last year, I had a minor operation. Because the antibiotics reacted seriously to my body, at one point I was sleeping at night, my whole body was half numb, I had a headache and could not sleep, it was painful. PL really helped me a lot, especially in emergencies, I felt not good enough to stick with it for a long time.

Later, I enrolled in a mindfulness class in January. After a few rounds of Paida on my arms and legs, the problem of numbness in my sleep was basically solved. During this period, there was another time. When I woke up in the morning, my feet were numb, so I immediately did Lajin in bed, the numbness in my feet cleared up soon. I really felt the magic of PL, tasted the sweetness, and I wanted to continue.

Afterwards, I wanted to unblock my body on a deeper level, so I joined this Paida of overall body class. I really felt the magic of PL as I trained with the teacher and my Paida fellows everyday. Because of my own lack of determination, I was impressed and admired the plain perseverance of Ms. Liu Ying for so many years, with palm by palm, leading everyone to persist.

I have personally experienced the helplessness of modern medicine. In 2011, I had hyperthyroidism for the birth of a baby. At first, I saw a western doctor and took western medicine for a week, I had a rash all over my body, the doctor said that the allergy was severe with liver damage. At that time, Iodine 131 treatment was recommended, I learned that Iodine 131 is a radiation treatment, with great impact. Thus, I did not do it. Then, I switched to another hospital and the doctor gave me a different medication. After taking that medication, I still had drug induced liver damage and my hyperthyroidism did not fully recover. I stopped going to visit the hospital. In my experience, Western medicine cannot heal hyperthyroidism.

I had not really a major illness until last year. It was so painfull. It was an emergency and I had to have surgery, it was not fully healed, and the medication caused paraplegia. I kept thinking that "Why can not I get rid of a major illness and create a bunch of other illnesses? Human body is supposed to redeem itself through self-healing.

However, I have stumbled along the way. In the past, I might have wondered why I was so unfortunate and why I was sick. At present, through PL's philosophy of mindfulness and being exposed to practice myself, I know that it is all my own decision, that all illness is karmic and the cause came from me.

Simultaneously, I am grateful for a lot. There was an emergency every time, there were all kinds of good people and good methods to help me, so that I did not have to only choose Western medicine. Although the process was hard, I was lucky and I believed that the outcome will be good.

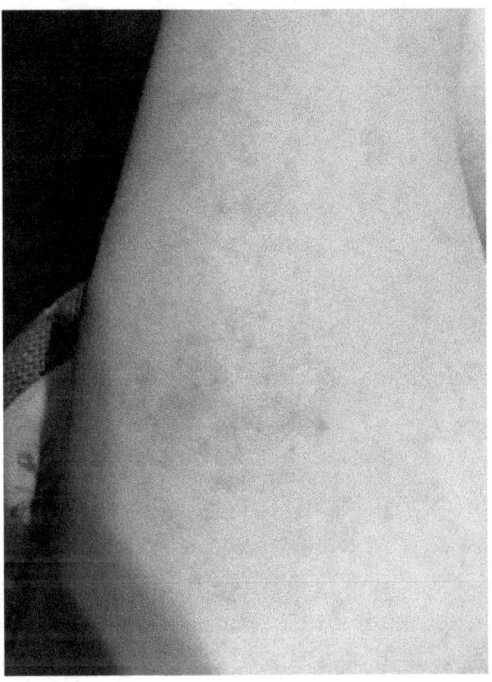

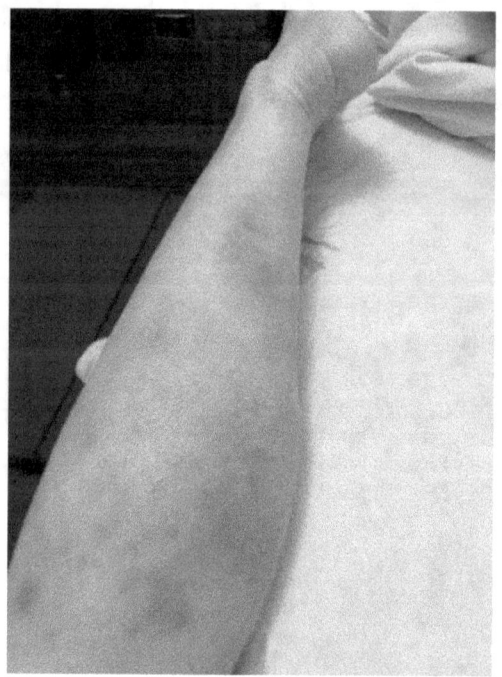

As I have benefited from it, I also want to spread and promote it to many people as possible. In the past, I had promoted it by taking a stretching bench and Paida tools to the elders' homes to pat at their home. I had patted the junior high school teachers and seriously ill colleagues, with the average effect. I felt that the main reason was that I was not persistent enough and I plan to get myself done well first. I should promote it with more confidence.

In addition, share again: it is good to pat the armpits, I had leaflet hyperplasia in my teens. I have visited to many hospitals, there was not healed. However, it was healed by Paida. It was so wonderful, whoever pat would know! I got well from patting my armpits plus breasts once at Paida camp in 2016 and have not had any pain since. Armpits were thick in the past, which was flat by Paida. I also had breast nodules in the pass, which was healed by Paida!

I would share another case. Last year, I was given a few days of antibiotics after surgery. My whole body was not in good condition, with serious mastitis in hard texture, it was very painful. At that time, the breast was too pain to Paida, I did Paida myself on two inner arms, it was healed by Paida for a few days.

The armpits and breasts of Paida are painful. Sisters, please bear it, the process is painful and the result is good.

My body is ssensitive now. After all these years, I also generally understand some Chinese medical concepts. The other day, as soon as I took intravenous injections at the hospital, I noticed something was wrong and my breasts started to swell and pain. I asked the little nurse, and she told me that do not overthink, it is funny! It shall always keep thinking about modern medicine.

Because the intravenous injection was conducted on my left side, my left eyelid was so swollen that I could not close it and it took two days to heal. Then I went home from hospital and slept at night and my whole left side went numb.

I read an article the other day that said if you take intravenous injections or have blood drawn, do not choose your left hand because your heart is on the left. It makes sense!

Most modern women have the problem, the root cause comes from emotions, stress and diet, nine of ten women have problems with their breasts, lobules, nodules and others. Unfortunately, many people will not accept it if you tell them about Paida.

Besides, the function on the groin of Paida was amazing. I shared it at the last mindfulness class. Because I was given the intravenous injections after surgery last year. When a bad vaginitis flared up, which had never been bad. I usually suffered from vaginitis too, with a little itchy. However, it was so intense at this time: severe itching and pain. Then I desperately patted the groin and the base of the thigh for a few days. Then, I discharged the exudation as thick as a wet napkin in the toilet. I was shocked at the time, then I thought it was a good thing, it returned to normal. At present, it is still slightly itchy, so I will continue to Paida.

Everything is in balance. If you give up the pain in your body and you get a healthy body in return. Thank you, I have finished my sharing here for today. Thanks for your precious time. Thanks for PL team, Coach Liu Ying for your persistence always, thank you!

-- Ms. Liu 2021.6.3

I had to read this report several times and cross-reference it before I could finally make some sense of the author's account, especially the "minor surgery" that she mentions several times. She is not ambiguous about one thing, i.e., is that she only comes up with PL when she is desperate. When she gets better, she forgets about it, and remembers it again at the next time she gets worse. She is indeed lovely in her frankness; we could have a glimpse of the 'dangerous game' in her clinical trials.

The root of her illness started from hyperthyroidism. "I experienced the helplessness of modern medicine for getting hyperthyroidism caused by having a baby in 2011." How could having a baby trigger hyperthyroidism? Hyperthyroidism can only be triggered by depression, so I can only guess that she was suffering from postnatal depression, or at least a bad mood. "First, she visited a Western doctor and took Western medicine for a week, had a rash all over her body and the doctor said she had severe allergies with liver damage. Iodine 131 treatment was recommended at the time, I learned that iodine 131 is a radioactive treatment with a high impact, so I did not receive the treatment." The aftermath of two radioactive treatments for hyperthyroidism in Indonesia in the previous case was disastrous and can be referred to. "The doctor gave me a different medication. After taking it, I still had drug-related liver damage and my hyperthyroidism was not completely healed. Then I stopped going to the doctor. In my experience, Western medicine has no solution for hyperthyroidism." Since I had read more cases, I realized why many hyperthyroid patients have bulging eyes, which is a consequence of medication damage to the liver. Because the liver is related to the eyes.

By 2016, her physical examination revealed four bad tumor indicators. She remembered to PL method, which she had learned about a few years earlier without doing it seriously. "At the 7-day camp, it was still fresh in my mind, it renewed a lot of my perceptions...After 7-days training and roughly 6 months of Paida at home, I went for a review, which indicated that 2 of 4 indicators had improved and other 2 indicator had dropped a lot, without taking any medication. PL was real and effective." There was little doubt that if she had used Paida treatment when she was first diagnosed with hyperthyroidism, she would have completely healed herself. Unfortunately, she did not have enough faith. Waiting for the cancer indicators to get bad before remembering PL was based on the Western clinical experience already experienced. It is the "dangerous game" of waiting for the disease to get worse before taking it seriously. Is not PL very effective? It should be integrated into your life and become a way of life!

However, "When they get better, they start to get lazy. In the following years, I occasionally conducted Paida and really did not do enough, "At the end of last year I had a minor operation. Because the antibiotics reacted seriously to my body. Once when I was sleeping at night, my whole body was half numb, I had a headache and could not sleep, it was painful. PL really helped me a lot, especially in emergencies, I felt really not good enough to stick with it for a long time." She stops here. It was only later that she recounted the "emergency": after a few days of intravenous injections of antibiotics after the operation last year, I was in a bad condition, my mastitis was bad, which was hard, it was painful. At that time, the breast was too pain with Paida, I did Paida myself on two inner arms, it was healed by Paida for a few days." I do not understand that why she did not pat on it earlier and waited for the disease to intensify before she remembered. What is even more puzzling is that "At the other day, as soon as taking intravenous injections at the hospital, I noticed something was wrong and my breasts started to swell and hurt. I asked the nurse, and she told me that do not overthink." Why did she take intravenous injections of antibiotics for a few days anyway if she already felt something was wrong? It shows where her confidence lies.

Did she say that PL would help her a lot in an emergency? Apparently, it was not urgent enough, and it was not until the post-operative drip caused her breasts to become massively painful in the hard texture, so that she finally thought about PL. Frankly, what she thought was a non-surgical condition was most efficiently resolved by Paida. You will find the various emergency cases in the *Emergency Clinical Report of PL*.

It can be concluded that PL is too simple, while the human heart is too complex. Therefore, her entire medical history and clinical experiments are a narrative of her mind that has been guided and changed by Western clinical and PL clinical. All clinical experiments seem to be a heal. In fact, they are regulating the mind and healing the heart. Hopefully, PL has really been integrated into the author's life. The "dangerous game" can be changed into a "happy and safe game".

## 1-20 Is her illness hyperthyroidism or heart disease?

I am a student of the ninth seven-day experience class in Shenzhen, I have been taking medicine for more than 20 years due to endocrine disorders, and I have been looking for external treatments of Chinese medicine to help me treat diseases for a long time. Once I accidentally saw Mr. Xiao's lecture on the Internet for introducing PL, which was what I wanted. Thus, I started to Paida and watched it. In less than a minute, a string of purple and black bruises came out. Later, I continued Paida on overall body and realized that my meridians were almost completely blocked, to completely unblock my meridians, I systematically learned PL method, and distanced myself from the hospital, I signed up for a seven-day experience class.

I knew before I came that I would have to do three days of fasting, which was a test for me. I had hyperthyroidism and the symptoms of the disease are easy hunger, shaky hands, rapid heartbeat, chest tightness and weight loss; even when my hyperthyroidism had been improved, I had to take maintenance medication. I stopped taking my medication the day I reported for the class (my lab results were normal in May). However, I was not steady, I had no idea if I would have to run and do PL in the morning when I am hungry, I did not know consuming so much the physical strength if I could handle it. As a result, from the day I started fasting, my pulse rate was 105/min. When I was at rest, I felt that my heart seemed to jump out of my chest and uncomfortable. When I felt uncomfortable, I followed the instructor's instructions and did Lajin the relevant areas. There were no other symptoms during the class, except for a rapid heartbeat. The day after the ending of camp, I accidentally took my pulse (after replenishing some energy) and found that it was normal. I could not believe the fact, so I counted it several times. My friends and family also verified that it was true. I was so happy! I realized that all illnesses were caused by blocked meridians, all illnesses will disappear along with the clear meridians. Through the seven days of experience, although my whole body was full of bruises, I had lost weight, the melanin on my face became lighter, my physical discomfort was improved, my body and mind had been baptized and tested, and I felt more refreshed and happy.

At the two hours after the end of the experience class, I was already patting with relatives and friends. After returning, my friends changed from bystanders to executors. My mother was so encouraged by the lecture that she stretched more and told me where she was uncomfortable, asked me to pat for her. The effectiveness of PL is shown! Thanks, Mr. Xiao and instructors! Specially, I am grateful to mommy of Mr. Xiao! An 70-year-old woman, who runs with the group every morning for exercise and works as a coach to guide and assist us in PL. I admired that she kept her energy up all the time, and she loaded three sandbags for Lajin.

-- Participant from the 9th Shenzhen Camp: Ms. Wang; September 14, 2011

Additional information: Ms. Wang came from Guangzhou, 52 years old, with hyperthyroidism for over 20 years. She had a pale face at the beginning. After a few days of practice, she was covered in bruises toxins from Paida and restored great spirits. Thank you for sharing her story. As a result, we have an enthusiastic PL health ambassador. We would wish Ms. Wang a speedy and complete recovery! Thank you Ms. Wang for introducing PL to more destined people!

-- Coach Qiu Jin; September 14, 2011

Looking at her symptoms: she was easy to hunger, with shaking hands, rapid heartbeat, chest tightness and weight loss, which were almost all symptoms of heart disease. In fact, the name heart disease should not be attached. To be more precise, it should be the blockage from the 6 meridians of the heart, pericardium, lungs, large intestine, small intestine and Tri-jiao, which are located on the front and back of the arm: three Yin meridians lead to the chest and three Yang meridians lead to the head and abdomen. Among above 6 meridians, the heart meridian is the most dominant and has the greatest influence on the symptoms, followed by the lung and large intestine meridians. As the lungs and the large intestine is cognate, they can be damaged relatively. The lungs are responsible for the exchange of gases inside and outside the body, while the intestines are responsible for food intake and detoxification, as well as the metabolic exchange inside and outside the body. Therefore, the heart, lungs and intestines are dysfunctional, people cannot absorb nutrients and detoxify normally, so that they are always in a state of fatigue, they are prone to hunger, trembling, and emaciation.

However, the biomarkers must be used to confirm the name of the disease in order to treat it in Western medicine. Blood pressure, blood sugar and thyroid can be measured, which can be easy to confirm the diagnosis. However, heart disease is difficult to diagnose. It is also the reason that heart disease is the leading cause of sudden and slow death worldwide. In this clinical case, for example, the description of the symptoms of the disease requires the use of indicators, called "endocrine disorder on medication for over 20 years", followed by "maintenance medication even if hyperthyroidism has been improved." If you ask a follow-up question: why is there an endocrine disorder? It is the cause of the disease and the key to heal the disease. However, the medicine is ignorant of it. The causes of almost all chronic diseases are unknown and it is unresolved. Therefore, the drugs are used to keep the normal indicators, which could mask the cause and create more illnesses.

A sentence that may be overwhelming is sited: the heart is the body's largest immune organ! The system associated with the heart is therefore the largest immune system. How does the heart function properly? It is by keeping the meridians associated with it open, specifically the 12 main meridians of the body, which shall be open for them to act properly. There are a few meridians that are more relevant and more important to keep open, namely the heart, lung, pericardium and large intestine meridians. These meridians are located on the arms and hands, which are the first parts of the body to do Lajin in the general area. How can the above statement be verified? The author attended a seven-day workshop to verify the diagnosis in a clinical setting.

At the end of the camp, she "accidentally took my pulse (after replenishing some energy) and found that it was normal. I could not believe the fact, so I counted it several times. My friends and family also verified that it was true. I was so happy!" It means that after more than 20 years of taking medication, her pulse was instead abnormal, and she had already got used to it being abnormal. Thus, she could not believe it was true. Why did she have a high pulse at the beginning of fasting? Because it was HC. Previously, its functions were controlled by external substances such as drugs and food. It was regulated by the internal Qi. It is reasonable to say that she already had easy hunger, shivering and symptoms. If it is not worse for three days of fasting? However, "no other symptoms appeared during this period, except for a rapid heartbeat." Even the symptom of a rapid heartbeat turned out to be a huge improvement later. Because HC are the diagnosis as well as the self-healing. It was HC that dissolved the worst of her symptoms for over 20 years. In other words, the worst illness healed by herself was heart disease, which was the general root cause of her hyperthyroidism and other illnesses.

She recalled her recent Paida by herself as below, "Once I accidentally saw Mr. Xiao's lecture for introducing PL on the Internet, which was just what I wanted, so I started to Paida during watching it. In less than a minute, a string of purple and black bruises came out. Later, I continued Paida of overall body and realized that my meridians were almost completely blocked." It was the root cause of her endocrine disorder for over 20 years: her meridians were not working. She was taking medication for years to boost her immune system. However, it was lowered. Because the toxins were further blocking her meridians, and the blocked meridians were the root cause of the immune system decline and naturally became the cause of all her illnesses. The blocked meridians refer to many functional disorders, in other words, reduction of immunity. The function of immunity depends on the open degree of the meridians. The causes of so-called endocrine disorders were often attributed to immune dysfunction, while the reason for the disorder was unknown. It has been clinically proven that the disorder is caused by the blocked meridians. If the meridians are opened by PL, the function gradually returns to normal. It is the same status for thyroid function as well as insulin, prostate and other endocrine functions.

Since the symptoms she listed were the most prominent in her heart disease, it was clear that her worst illness was heart disease. Thus, her symptoms would be resolved, Her heartbeat and chest congestion would naturally improve by opening up the heart, pericardium and lung meridians; her digestive function would improve and her nutrient absorption would be normalized by Paida on the large intestine, small intestine and Tri-jiao meridians on the other side of her arm, so that her hunger and shakiness would also improve. The healing not only focuses on the disease, the name of the disease, or the indicator, but also on the blockage of the meridians that caused the disease. Her body was covered in bruises after attending the camp, with a manifestation of the detoxification of the meridians, which resulted in the weight loss, lighter melanin on her face, improved the physical discomfort and "a feeling of well-being and happiness." It is the healing effect of PL instead of medicine. It also proves that the heart is the largest immune organ of body. She actually had heart disease. The rest of her illnesses were merely complications of heart disease.

## 1-21 Hyperthyroidism sequelae and heart disease and cardiopathy

Hello, everyone! My name is Xiao Hui. I am glad to have the opportunity to share my experience of PL with you, today.

I came across PL in 2014 when I was trying to find a good way to stay fit and healthy. After a brief study and understanding, I bought the necessary tools and started practising. At that time, I was in the stage of practicing blindly. I felt that I had achieved my goal when the bruises came out by Lajin. Although it was blind, it was effective. Thus, I recommended PL to my family and friends. Some of them questioned the effectiveness of PL, said that it would break blood vessels, that it was unscientific and other criticisms. However, I was not swayed.

I was convinced by PL's theory that "If your tendons grow by an inch, your life expectancy will increase by 10 years" and "Blockage accompanies pain, non-blockage refer to no pain".

In 2015, I attended a beginner's course and learned a lot. It was like a guerrilla meeting a regular army. I started to learn more systematically PL method, the auxiliary gong methods and the foot soaking and grain removal methods. My physical condition has improved greatly. I could also have more confidence in PL.

I lost my weight, had more energy and felt better in every aspect of my body. Thus, inertia slowly took over too, I had less frequent of PL and dragging out a lot of days.

I started feeling unwell again in 2018, often lacking energy. I knew that I had to act. However, I always unable to make up my mind. It just likes as procrastination, it is not hurry until the deadline. Thus, it was until the beginning of last year when I finally felt I had to make a change, and taking a carpet class was the start of a real change for me. It was a two-hour PL everyday, which was tiring. I hardly took a break, and I took my daily tasks seriously. Because I knew that I had to get my health back by PL.

During Paida, I had HC, with a daily headache that lasted for a whole week. The headaches were an old problem of mine, the aftermath of hyperthyroidism. It hurts so often, which was painful. After the carpet class, although it was not healed, the headaches were significantly no more frequent. The physique has also increased. I mastered PL again, the magic weapon of strengthening my body. I told myself that I could not lose it again.

I felt that it was enjoyable to follow the teacher to Paida. Coach Liu has a good mid-range and a loud voice, with the right rhythm, which did not get tired easily. Especially when you do not know the method of Paida, watch the action of the instructor. Whether it is posture, angle or strength, you can copy it.

I signed up for the Manipulative Mindfulness class again in March this year, a worthwhile Paida class where the instructor shared all her years of Paida experience, which was beneficial. Each move seems simple and yet not simple, there is a method and a way in it, you must take your time to experience it. Once you have embodied it, you could improve and double the effect of PL. After the mmindfulness class, I could not wait to sign up for the carpet class again this term. You will only know how good your choice is if you take it! It was blissful to have something you look forward to everyday. It was especially surprising that you could feel better sleep, lighter body, finer skin and others after Paida.

Experiences about PL

1. As for Paida: I feel that Paida with our hands is more conducive to communicating with all parts of our body than Paida with tools. Professor Zeng Shiqiang once spoke about his own communication with the body, which inspired me. Our bodies have served us for so many years. We think more about that how we feel and ignore what the body itself can take. Asking for too many causes the body to become overdrawn. When we do Paida with our hands, the Laogong acupoint (an acupoint on the hear meridian) on the palm of our hands represents our hearts, and its contact with the part is communicateded with Lajin. The warmth strength and softness of our hands are more easily accepted by our body compared to tools and combined with our words (four aphorisms or sincere repentance) or intentions (health/illness

removed/dispersed and others), the effect of Paida will be twice as effective.

2. About pain: I have improved my understanding of pain in the manipulative mmindfulness class. When you focus on the area being Paida and think of your debt to it, your heart became soft and compassionate, you will not clench for fear of pain, and your muscles can be relaxed at this time. The pain is lessened by Paida in this way. I felt less like I was in pain and sucking in my breath the time in the carpet class. Basically, every slap was accurate. Focused, relaxed, rhythmic Paida was not tiring. Especially when patting blindfolded, as the instructor said, it reduces distraction and helps Paida to be more productive. In fact, there are many times when we feel tired. Because we have too many distractions and consume a lot of energy. During the mindfulness class, I not only did PL, but also went to play ball with friends and did housework without any delay. The pace of life was not even affected, so that I did not hesitate to enroll in the carpet class.

3. About Lajin (stretching): What I did the most were lying Lajin, Lajin with stretching board and squat Lajin. The changes that have been brought to my body are better flexibility, lighter walking legs. I have the urge to run when I walk after Lajin for a few days. My friends said that I was in a youthful state. I would like to share with you that "if you keep going a little longer, you might get a surprise". Every time I stand on the stretching board, I find the hardest time for keeping 25 minutes of standing stretching board, my arms are numb and my heels are aching, so that I want to get off. However, once I held on for another five minutes, it was surprised that my numb left hand regained its sensation, we had removed and ceased the bruises by Paida. Later, when I stood on the stretching board again, I had to hold on for a longer time when my hand was numb. Maybe I do not have the frozen shoulders that people should have this disease at my age for the perseverance. In fact, it is the same with other stretches, you can feel a really difference that you can not go on for another 5 minutes every time.

4. About foot soaking and fasting: it is no denying that two regimens are all very good. It is said that for every degree of increase in human body temperature, the immune system

improves by 15%. The best way to raise your body temperature shall soak your feet until you became sweaty a little. Please do not sweat a lot, it is easy to be weak. I soak two or three times a week and my feet are always warm. Warmness is proof that Qi and blood can get to them with the open meridians. It is the credit of the foot soak.

I also agree with the idea of incantation, while the duration of incantation should vary from person to person and should not be forced. I once tried one day a week for six months and felt fine, my spleen and stomach had time to rest and I was not too tired. My weight was stable, around 55kg. I had also tried 3 days a month, which can test the endurance. You shall not be moved in front of the food, as soon as the heart wants to eat, the stomach will be conditioned to squirm digestion, it is easy to hurt the stomach. Secondly, please do not feel that you have no energy if you do not eat. You shall believe that your stored energy can get you through 3-day fasting. However, it is a personal experience and each individual is different, so you should prepare your body and mind before you do PL. Otherwise, the benefits will not be worth the losses.

It has been 8 years since I learned about PL. By reflecting on my performance, I was just lazy and procrastinating. I had decided that I could participate in the various resonance classes of Coach Liu when I am lazy again, so that the great energy field of resonance can bring me strength.

I am grateful to have come across such a good fitness method! I am grateful to have met such a good coach and her team! I am grateful to meet all of you! I would hope that everyone will take PL as their daily nutritional meal to achieve true self-health! Have a happy life! Thank you!

--Xiao Hui, 2022.5.3

Two sequelae of hyperthyroid were mentioned in the report: headache and insomnia. In fact, these are symptoms of heart disease, which are the result of blockages in the heart and pericardium meridians. If we dig deeper, we will find that thyroid disease is the result of blockage of the heart, pericardium, lung and large intestine meridians. Headaches, insomnia, panic attacks, weakness and other symptoms are also symptoms of blockages in these meridians, except that people can feel them, which is different as thyroid, where the specific biological indicators can be identified.

Among these blocked meridians, the heart and pericardial meridians are the most important, as the function of the heart depends on their smoothness. What causes the heart and pericardial meridians to be incompetent? Heart disease stems from mainly negative emotions and false perceptions, which is more deeply hidden than negative emotions. Her hyperthyroidism was caused by her heart disease, which was not detailed in the text. We can find out the cause of the disease and the root of the condition at least from the heart disease that was implicitly revealed in her healing process.

She took the class for beginner in 2015 and "my health was improved a lot; I could have more confidence about PL. I lost my weight, had more energy, and felt better in every aspect of my body. Thus, inertia slowly took over, she had less PL frequently and dragging out a lot of days." It was IIC of heart disease. The word of inertia has a vertical heart side (in Chinese), which expressed the fact that the root of this state stems from the heart. The state of mind showed that PL had not really entered her heart. However, it is merely a "rudimentary" remedy for a temporary emergency. The mentality is like the condition of the previous writer, which is also the mentality of many Paida fellows. Bluntly speaking, she has a lot of things to do that are more important than Paida. PL and the body are tools used by people, their specific application depends only on the heart. What appears to be "inertia" is laziness in fact that stems from human knowledge. Because PL is not yet important in her system of thought and values, there are so many great causes, goals and the enjoyable things in life to strive for! PL could only reappear in her life when her condition was deteriorated. It is the "dangerous game".

Certainly, " I started feeling unwell again in 2018, often lacking energy in 2018." The weakness is a symptom of a blocked heart meridian, rather than a symptom of hyperthyroidism. "I knew that I had to act. While I am always unable to make up my mind." It is heart disease. Heart disease and cardiac disease are manifested by blockages in the heart, pericardium and lung meridians. You will know the performance of PL! "Thus, it was until the beginning of last year (i.e. 2020) when I finally felt I had to make a change, and taking a carpet class was the start of a real change for me.." That's why I joined the carpet class (i.e. Paida of the whole body)." I had HC during Paida and had daily headaches lasting for a whole week. The headaches were an old problem of mine, a sequel to hyperthyroidism." If it is an old problem, why do not you completely dissolve it by PL? Hyperthyroidism is just a name for a disease and headache is just a symptom. Since it has been untreated for years, the cause of the disease has not been found. After Paida of the inside and outside of the arm and the head, I had been feeling better! It is so simple. Certainly, "I was not healed in the carpet class, but the headaches were significantly less frequent. The physique has also increased. I got back to PL as a magic tool for strengthening my body." She later attended the mindfulness class and was "pleasantly surprised by the improved sleep, the lightness of her body, the refinement of her skin and others." These are still the symptoms that improved after opening up the heart meridian. All improvements in heart disease were just caused by a new decision made by her heart. The heart is the master, that is what it means.

There are four experiences of PL that she summed up all their experiences of mindfulness.

1. About Paida: she talks about communicating with the body by hand, tools and words. In fact, communication between the mind and the body is emphasized.
2. About pain: It is more of a major shift in the mind, i.e. a change in the interpretation of pain. Although you are still dealing with pain, a phenomenon, your interpretation about it is something that you can re-choose by your mind. If you treat it as an enemy, you will naturally have a completely different effect than that if you treat it as a friend; it is same to the body. Reinterpreting the phenomenon refers to the change of knowledge.

3. About Lajin: it is still your interpretation of pain and numbness, that is, the attitude of your mind, that determines the effect.
4. About foot soaking and fasting: whether you agree with them and implement them depends on your knowledge and confidence. The knowledge can be learned. However, confidence must be built through experiences. Whether you learn or not depends on your heart, and experience can only be experienced by the mind. This auxiliary Paida methods are the same as Paida, which can only be learned through experience in the clinic. It depends on the heart.

Thus, the self-healing from hyperthyroidism is self-healing from heart disease. Furthermore, the heart is regulated and healed in the process. Once the heart is regulated at peace, the heart disease can be resolved. Moreover, the other complications, such as thyroid disease, can also be naturally resolved.

## 1-22 The sequelae of thyroid cancer self-heals

I am a person with many diseases. Although PL process was slow to take effect. There were no immediate results (as I was a long and strenuous worker, I retired and learned about PL in my sixties). However, the body did improve considerably.

**Health status before PL:**

I was a thyroid cancer patient and it had spread to two lymph and received a total thyroid removal surgery in March, 2017. Six months after the operation, I suddenly developed mild cataracts in both eyes, which were so severe: a thick fog in front of my eyes, inability to see light and rapid vision loss that I finally opted for cataract removal in both eyes.

In the past, I was so weak that I could not walk, my appetite was very poor, my bowels were not formed for a long time, my internal and external hemorrhoids were itchy, I had a cold frequently, poor sleep at night and other major and minor discomforts, even I thought my life was coming to an end.

Improvements:

Through the daily practices of PL, all these symptoms have improved to various degrees.

The biggest change has been in my spirit. In the past, I was reluctant to do anything and was too lazy to even talk due to lack of energy. Whenever I heard that a colleague or friend was coming to visit me, I was afraid. Because I had no energy to receive them. Due to my laziness, I had to buy the children's breakfast everyday, and the thought of going downstairs was a heavy burden.

Now, I take it upon myself to do all the general household chores. For breakfast, I make my own porridge, buns, pancakes or other fancy snacks. It's no problem to walk outside for an hour or two hours. everyday I pick up my child from the kindergarten 20 minutes away from home and accompany him to the educational institution. I said to my daughter, "If I am willing to do something, that means I am still fit. If I do not want to move, it must be something wrong with my body".

How do I PL? I came to know about the self-healing method when I entered PL's public account after a friend posted a picture of alleviating back and leg pain in old age. After reading some case studies shared, I followed to do Paida on my own. Since I was in poor health, I got started without studying Theory totally.

I did PL everyday slowly, bruises were not coming out, if I have a warm feeling. Everything is changed unintentionally. I must pat my head and face for an hour and a half everyday with the numerous benefits: my mind will be clear, my vision and hearing will be enhanced.

**Did you experience HC during Paida? Were you consistent to Lajin?**

Because of the changes in my body, I started to believe in PL. However, it was a sudden change in my eyes, PL was stopped, and my psychophysics went to the freezing point. Later, I still started PL, and tried to learn from the instructors, volunteers, and experienced seniors in Paida group, to do PL correctly and avoid detours, so that the current effect was gained.

There was no other noticeable HC except for eye problems, maybe I was insensitive. I did Lajin everyday for short time. Because, I must manage the kids and do housework. Recently, I have stopped lying Lajin (I would love to do them). However, I have done M-Lajin for more than half an hour everyday (mainly for my gut), and I chose to Y-shape Lajin or neck Lajin. I'm still going to add lying Lajin everyday.

I have not taken any more medication or supplements since I got sick and had the operation, apart from the Eugenol which I had to take. I still shall keep trying to learn from my friends and adjust my mental and physical state, so that I can live a healthy life. Thus, PL is effective. We shall believe in PL and perist in it.

-- Yansha Mengxing, March 3, 2019

The so-called thyroid cancer is essentially no different from other thyroid diseases. Therefore, the sequelae are no different either, it is mainly the result of blockages in the heart, pericardium, lung and large intestine meridians. The symptoms of blockage of the central and pericardial meridians are the worst: too weak to be able to walk, "I was reluctant to do anything and was too lazy to even talk due to lack of energy" due to weakness", I had a cold frequently and had poor sleep at night." The large intestine meridian and the lung meridian is mutually relative, so her symptoms can be considered as one category, which is mainly unformed stools, itchy internal and external hemorrhoids. Itchiness can also be considered as a type of skin disease, while the lung dominates the skin. The cataracts in both eyes were caused by the damage to the liver, as the liver is the master of the eyes. Most of the liver damage is caused by the negative effects of the medication used in the treatment of hyperthyroidism. We have seen several cases of liver damage from taking medication.

As a result of PL, "All symptoms improved to varying degrees. The biggest change has been in my spirit. In the past, I was reluctant to do anything and too lazy to even talk due to lack of energy. Whenever I heard that a colleague or friend was coming to visit me, I was afraid because I had no energy to receive them. At present, I take the initiative to do all the household chores. For breakfast, I made porridge, steamed buns and pancakes. It is no problem to walk outside for an hour or two hours."

It is evident that the greatest improvements are in the heart and intestines, the result of the opening of the heart, pericardium, lung and large intestine meridians. The simplest question was raised from the clinical result: since weakness, indigestion and other symptoms were judged to cause thyroid imbalance, the thyroid gland was completely removed, and Eugenol has been taken to regulate thyroid secretion. Why did these symptoms not improve? Why did all the symptoms improve so dramatically after PL, especially the severe weakness? It became clear whether the improvement in her weakness and mental health was caused by the Qi activated by the opening of the meridians or the medicinal power obtained by taking Eugenol. Whether a person gains energy directly from the opening of the meridians, or gains Qi and nutrition from the improved functions of the heart and thyroid after opening meridians, it is the result of opening the meridians, especially the heart, pericardium, lung, and large intestine meridians. Although her thyroid gland was completely removed, did these improvements prove that the thyroid function was still partially restored after PL through the meridians? The fact has been shown from the clinical findings. If it is not, why did she not achieve improvement on Eugenol? If you are still in doubt about PL, please read the next clinical report.

Talking about her specific clinical course, she mentioned that she had stopped the patches because of a sudden change in her eyes and "my psychophysics went to freezing point. Later, I still started PL, and tried to learn from the instructors, volunteers and experienced seniors in Paida group, to do PL correctly with fewer detours. So that the current effect was gained." She was obviously frightened by HC, and it was related to the fact that she "got started without studying Theory totally". Many people are too scared to do it. Because they do not understand HC at first and take it as a bad thing. Therefore, it is important to learn as much as possible about the fundamentals before patting to build confidence and implement Paida. It is also important to join a Paida group as it is a great treasure trove for learning about mindfulness and technique. If she could join camp and do several Paida of full body, she would be able to take her body and mind to the next level.

She also said, "I did Lajin everyday for short time. Because, I have to manage the kids and do housework. Recently, I have stopped lying Lajin (I would love to do them)." That's anxiety all over again! And it's a serious anxiety. Why is that? Because it fully revealed her inner knowing, i.e. her mind, her value system. We could image that how miserable she was when she was so sick that she was unable to speak or receive friends! When her body had recovered a little, the time for healing was gone, the time and energy for creating illness was gone! It is only natural to work for your family. If you are a sick person who has not yet recovered, why not heal your illness first before you work on your household? It can be concluded that the reason for her previous illness was related to this knowledge and insight: overworking for the extremely important things that she considered. Whether you are overworking for your career, your family, or anything, illness will be caused by your misconception. Because the purpose of your struggle is not to die early. Once you understand that your daily business and habits are creating diseases and accelerating death, you will naturally correct your perceptions and goals and reduce the obstacles in your heart. Otherwise, the heart meridian and pericardial meridian will be blocked. Thus, starting from heart disease, these complications emerge one after another. She has not healed yet she was too busy to Lajin!

Thus, the sequelae of thyroid cancer that she healed herself by PL were her old illnesses actually: anxiety and heart disease. Hyperthyroidism and thyroid cancer are just symptoms of anxiety and heart disease. If her energy and spirit is just recovered, her mind and her knowledge is not changed, her behaviour and habits will immediately return to the old patterns, i.e. the disease is sometimes created. However, there is no time for self-healing. It is noteworthy that she said, "I did not do lying Lajin anymore, while I wanted to do it actually." It is a conflict between old and new knowledge, which means that the heart disease is still existing in HC. Whether she is so busy that she does not even have time to heal herself is really a matter of her thoughts. The fate of the body is actually determined by this thought.

## 1-23 PL's recovery from thyroid cancer

Hello, Mr. Xiao!

I happened to have a relationship with Ms. Gaoshan (Teacher Zhao Ruihua) and naturally with PL. I am a cautious person. Although I believed in PL the first time I came into contact with it but I will only recommend it to others if I have good results myself. The exception was this time. I had only started PL for a few days and recommended it to my sister, who has thyroid cancer. What I felt was pain and nothing else was gained. A month later, I went for a review. I was truly surprised to witness that my sister had made a full recovery. Her removed thyroid gland had regenerated and was still healthy. In response to the encouragement from the group, I wrote about my sister's case to share with friends who are destined. Perhaps a spark of hope can be ignited for other people in the same situation.

My sister had been diagnosed with thyroid nodules before and had concerns about them. A few months ago, the thyroid nodule grew rapidly and the doctor recommended surgery. Thus, she chose to go to XX Hospital in Chongqing for a partial excision. The specialist who operated at the time judged it to be benign, while the result was heartbreaking, and it was diagnosed as malignant. As the surgeon estimated that it was benign, she did not remove all of it during the operation. Once the result came out, it seemed that the part left was a bomb that would explode at any time, which can cause to her constant worry.

After her surgery, she was discharged from hospital and went home to recuperate without any radiotherapy or chemotherapy. When we went to visit her, we discussed the next steps in her treatment. From my point of view, firstly, we should not over-treat. Many cancer patients die faster only because they over-treat and cause further damage to their bodies. This view was agreed by my brother-in-law and sister. Secondly, it is not permitted to accept any folk remedies for poisonous insects and herbs. It is not certain whether they can heal the disease. However, it is certain that long-term consumption leads to chronic poisoning of the body. It was also agreed by brother-in-law and sister. Thirdly, the amount of cancer cells in my sister's body was the same as cancer cells in mine (I'm also saying it to release stress from her mind), and her masses that were more than mine have been cut out. She shall not overthink it. The cancer cells on me did not harm my body. Because my resistance was okay, and I was able to control it. My sister shall tune her body to the same level as mine and she will be able to control it. When my sister asked that how to do it, I gave her the first three-dimensional regimen that I had ever used in my life for cancer patients:

1. Choose moxibustion to warm up the meridians and disperse cold, to support Yang and strengthen the body. All acupuncture acupoints are related to strengthen the body only.
2. Do not be psychologically burdened, do not overthink and keep your mood relaxed.
3. Exercise properly;
4. Eat a reasonable diet, and add some food therapy schemes.

In fact, before I went here, my sister was already doing the last three items. Next, I added moxibustion into the treatment and went to push the primal points on her head and upper back and scrape her back from time to time. I also gave her hand-held moxibustion on her back when I went to scrape. A friend told me that hand-held moxibustion is more effective for major illnesses. I did not dare to tell her or show her that black bruises came out when I was scraping her back. I would not increase her psychological burden.

My sister also recognized these methods, and did calisthenics, dietary therapy and moxibustion step by step everyday. After almost two months of the treatment, her health was getting better. However, she went to Chongqing for a follow-up check-up after the surgery at the first time, her other conditions were fine, except that the adenoma had reappeared in the area where the surgery had been performed. Her attending doctor said that it was probably scar tissue from the surgery. It shall be checked again at her re-reviewing. We said that it was probably scar tissue for consoling her. In fact, our family was as apprehensive as her.

Afterwards, I encountered PL and was very approving. According to some Chinese medical practices I knew, Paida is a technique of scraping, and the acceptance of stretching stems from the original point. My sister and I do not live in the same place. Thus, I basically went to her place once a week to give her scraping, massage the primal points and do hand-held moxibustion. When I was not there, the moxibustion was conducted by the tool. Over a period, she felt an improvement in her original cold hands and feet. Moxibustion was better for her conditions. As her serious illness, there were too few opportunities for me to help her, the effectiveness of the conditioning on her body is compromised. Besides, if I must go to Shenzhen once, I am afraid that I will have to delay her physiotherapy treatment again. What can I do?

PL method came into my mind that I was experiencing. Besides, I had seen many successful cases of various kinds of illnesses on Mr. Xiao's blog. When I went to give my sister a treatment, I introduced PL method to her as well. She was taught to Paida the generic area first and other areas, leaving the surgical areas untouched. I believed that when I was away, at least her Paida would be equivalent to that I patted her with this method, she would get better results if she can pat herself everyday.

After returning from Shenzhen, I have been busy always and finally had the time to visit my sister. I had to admire her action. After she did Paida the general area, she did Paida for hours wherever she felt bloated, numb, and itchy. She did Paida her body during the daytime and at night. Basically, wherever she did Paida, the bruises would appear. (I did not expect to write a sharing article at that time. Thus, I did not take any photos.) Her hands broke the skin and bled repeatedly. As my sister's mobility was so strong, I bought Mr. Xiao's PL book on Taobao for her and told her to follow the WeChat platform of PL, so that she could do PL more correctly. She was also reinforced with many successful cases to strengthen her confidence in PL. Because it is more powerful for the patient to have confidence in herself than for us to have confidence and act.

My sister has become more active. After Paida, she stopped her aerobics and everything. Because Paida is exercise, it can also detoxify and remove stagnant blood. She also insists on soaking her feet by mugwort every night. At first, she only used Paida for a while. When I came back from Shenzhen to visit her, I taught her to do her first stretching again by a chair against the wall.. She was better than me, and the Y-shape Lajin was conducted for half an hour. She felt that no amount of stretching was as good as by stretching bench, so that she bought her own immediately. My sister became better from these green therapies. You cannot tell that she is a cancer patient from her appearance.

The time soon came again for the re-examination. As it was close to the New Year, it was a bit far to travel from Zhunyi to Chongqing, so my sister thought she would just have a review at the local hospital. The first result of the review indicated that her thyroid gland was in the same size on two sides and no abnormality was found. She did not believe it. As one side of her thyroid had been mostly cut out and only a small part of it was left. How could it be the same size? Either the hospital was wrong, or what she feared had happened - another tumor had grown. With the apprehension in mind, I went to Chongqing for a review and got the same results as the local hospital, the blood tests were normal, no problems were found, and the removed thyroid was indeed healthy and regenerating!

What a miracle! My sister's cancer was the focus of attention. She also had hypertension for many years. With some fitness regimes, her blood pressure was under control, she still had to take anti-hypertensive medication once every few days. At present, her blood pressure is also normal and she has stopped taking all medication. She has stopped drinking the difficult dietary soup and switched to ginger and date tea.

Yesterday, I went to my sister's house again to write this story. I saw that she had gained a little weight, her skin was better, and she said that she looked better after PL. She must be happy that she has gone from being a cancer patient to being a healthy person, and the family is happy too. Thus, PL has been accepted and promoted in my family without any doubt. At present, my sister is promoting PL method to her family and close friends, her book is being passed around. Two days ago, I ordered ten more books from the E-bay shop for my family to have a copy and we are talking about Paida. Even my 83-year-old mother has been active in PL, the family surprised the first results with their PL and they want to share it with other family members and friends!

Although my sister did not do with PL at first, the scraping that I used in the early days was the same principle as Paida. However, Paida is stronger and can expel toxins hidden inside the body deeply beyond scraping. After going through a few scrapes at the same area, the patient still feels pain and I can feel the bumps, while the bruises cannot come out. Because the scraping pad is not strong enough to tune out the deeper toxins. Whereas Paida is stronger, it can clear the deeper layers and unblock blood vessels strongly, the method is simple. Those friends who have endured bruises and Paida have chosen Paida. Since my sister has used Paida, I have not given her any more scrapes either. I helped her with Paida too. The method has also freed me up from visiting my sister's house frequently. If I was to come across another cancer patient, I would just do Paida instead of scraping again.

I was lucky to learn about PL method from Ms. Gaoshan and bring it to my family, so that they could get healthy. I was also lucky that my sister did not have any major HC during the whole treatment (there was no ups and downs of HC as other friends), she had farts and occasional small heart pains (she had suffered from myocarditis before), the minor pains can be ignored. When I asked her if she had any HC, she thought about it and said that she had not noticed anything other than that. We were fortunate enough to encounter PL and benefit from it. I am grateful to Mr.

Xiao for his kindness to all sentient beings under the sun, and those who are destined will benefit.

My friend said his viewpoint about my sister's case: Although the individual cases do not represent the whole picture, they can give hope to those patients with similar illnesses.

My sister's whole regimen was not one-dimensional; it was called as three-dimensional conditioning. It could be summarized as below:

(1) Condition the mind. Do not be burdened with thoughts. Forget the name of the disease. (It is mentioned both in the books and videos of Mr. Xiao)

(2) Condition and strengthen the body. Moxibustion is chosen (rotating acupuncture acupoints by moxibustion to strengthen the body: Zhongwan, Shenjue, Guangyuan, Qihai, Dazhui, Mingmen, Zusanli, Sanyinjiao and Yongquan acupoints)

(3) Adjust the disease. PL aims at all the big and small diseases in your body together, rather than a single disease.

(4) Food therapy. Dietary treatment: 60 g Hedyotis diffusa, 60 g hawthorn and 1 turtle (about 500g, the breeding or wild turtle could be fine) is stewed together, people can eat meat and soup. My sister made a snapper stewed twice with medicine, drank and ate it for three days. This recipe is suitable for all types of cancer.

I am grateful to Mr. Xiao, Ms. Gaoshan, Moxibustion, PL and everyone who shared their cases with us. All of you have shown us with the spark of hope, so that it is possible for me to have good stories to share with you, today. My family and I will also share PL method of self-healing and health with more friends around us. I hope that more people can know more about PL!

--Zunyi Seventh Brother, 2015.03.02

In the previous thyroid cancer case discussion, we have raised a question: Why did the patient is too weak to walk and too lazy to talk after her total thyroidectomy? While after PL, she became more energy to do household chores and walk outside for an hour or two hours without any problem. Why did not she have such effectiveness when she was taking Eugenol? Does it mean that PL has partially restored the thyroid function? Since the previous example only mentioned symptoms that improved significantly and did not go to hospital for examination, the results in this case provided exactly the clinical findings of the hospital examination: "My sister had made a full recovery. Even the removed thyroid gland had regenerated and was still healthy."

In fact, even the patient herself initially did not believe that she would achieve these good results. She was first examined at a local hospital in Zhunyi and the results showed that "both thyroid glands were the same size without any abnormalities. My sister did not believe it. As one side of her thyroid had been mostly cut out and only a small part was left. How could it be the same size? Either the hospital was wrong, or what she feared had happened - another tumor had grown. With the apprehension in mind, I went to Chongqing for a review and got the same results as the local hospital, the blood tests were normal, no problems were found and the removed thyroid was indeed healthy and regenerating!"

This clear clinical result recalled us what I have repeatedly stressed in many previous clinical discussions: the immune system disorders are meridian blockages; the various conditions of immune system are also caused by the meridian blockages; it can be further concluded that all inflammatory-type conditions and neurodegenerative conditions are also caused by the meridian blockages. In the series of blocked meridians, the heart, lung, and pericardium meridians are the most critical, followed by the large intestine, small intestine and Tri-jiao meridians. You can read more clinical cases and discussions in *Clinical Comparison of Pain and Depression*, *Clinical Report on Lung and Intestinal Disorders*, *Clinical Report on Lung and Respiratory Disorders*, and *Clinical Report on Lung and Skin Disorders*.

Another special feature of this report is that the author himself has long done clinical experiments with three other natural therapies, namely scraping (bruise), Primal Point and Moxibustion. Thus, he had to compare PL clinical with his own common methods. He wrote, "Although my sister did not do with PL at first, the scraping that I used in the early days was the same principle as Paida. However, Paida is stronger, which can tune out toxins hidden inside the body deeply beyond scraping. After going through a few scrapes at the same area, the patient still feels pain and I can feel the bumps, while the bruises can not come out. Because the scraping pad is not strong enough to tune out the deeper toxins. Whereas Paida is stronger, it can clear the deeper layers, the unblocks blood vessels more strongly, and the method is simple. Those friends who have endured bruises and Paida have chosen PL. Since my sister had used Paida, I have not given her any more scrapes either. I also helped her with Paida. The method has also freed me up from going to my sister's house frequently. If I was to come across another cancer patient, I would just do Paida instead of scraping again."

He mentions that scraping is not as strong as PL, which is only one aspect of the process, but also that the direction of force is different. Scraping is done on the surface of the body, whereas Paida is done vertically up and down. Thus, the penetration effect and strength is naturally different. The biggest difference is the use of mental force. Because Paida is a self-healing method, it is entirely up to one's own mind to decide. Even mutual Paida is decided by our own soul. The whole process of implementation with concentrated attention is better than use of force and technique. In fact, her sister's Paida was basically a clinical experiment done by herself.

The success of the patient's recovery is also evident from the clinical aspects of her PL, which is extremely simple, with fewer detours. People who are complex-minded or have too much knowledge always prefer to practice superficially or give up halfway, or they cannot practice deeper because of doubts, fear and other heart diseases. It is simple Paida method, which does not emphasize the complications of meridians and acupuncture points. Although we have to use a simple general knowledge of meridians in our discussions, I always say to Paida the universal parts first and then the whole body during teaching others. The universal areas refer to the limbs, as everyone knows. That's exactly her Paida method, "After she did Paida the general area, she did Paida for hours wherever she felt bloated, numb and itchy." It is so simple!

Everyone's patience with Paida varies greatly. She was "patting for many hours at one time basically, wherever she did Paida, the bruises would appear. Her hands broke the skin and bled over again." Some people are too frightened to pat when the skin breaks and bleeds. However, they do not know that it is HC when the skin bleeds or the patting hand blisters. It is HC, which detoxifies the meridians. The palms of the hands are also full of meridian points and the three meridians of the heart, lungs and pericardium are also on the hands, where being repeated stimulation will greatly unblock three meridians, the blockage is a direct cause of heart disease, cardiac disease, lung disease and thyroid disease. As for stretching, she initially used a chair against the wall, she "felt that the stretching can have better effectiveness by a stretching bench. Thus, she immediately bought a stretching bench." In conclusion, her success with stretching is simple and focused, and her dedication is the critical reason. Without the confidence and patience, there are a lot of reasons why you can not do it properly for long term. Thoughts reside in the mind and operate in accordance with the instructions of the mind, which is the source of healing.

Whenever I say that all illnesses are complications of heart disease, many people are not convinced. This case is a clear clinical validation that: "My sister's cancer was the main focus of attention, but she also had hypertension for many years... At present, her blood pressure is also normal and she is completely off her medication. The original difficult therapeutic soup is no longer being consumed and has been replaced by ginger and date tea." What is hypertension? It's a symptom of heart disease, which is the same as insomnia, headaches, and others. How do you prove it? Paida on the heart and pericardium meridians the treatment is done simultaneously. It can be explained bluntly: hypertension, thyroid disease, cancer, insomnia, headaches, and other symptoms are all different ways of manifesting heart disease. Because cancer, hypertension, thyroid, and other diseases have indicators to confirm and show changes that human healing always revolves around these symptoms with indicators and ignores or does not know the cause of these diseases: blocked meridians, and the first meridians to be blocked are the heart meridian and pericardium meridian, which is the heart disease.

Some people may ask: if it is other cancers, such as lung cancer, liver cancer, gallbladder cancer, colon cancer and others, how should I do PL? Answer: it is the same as this case, pat the general area and the whole body, combined with the stretching. Another person asks: If it is another serious disease, such as dementia, hypertension, kidney failure, diabetes, skin disease, gynecological disease, neurodegenerative disease, other autoimmune system diseases and others. How to do PL? There is the same answer. The names of diseases change, they are all different manifestations of meridian blockages. Cancer is just an artificial name for a type of disease.

The question and answer above could be considered a reply to the comment mentioned in the article, "The individual cases do not represent the whole picture, but they can give hope to those with similar illnesses." It may sound like a positive statement. In fact, it is already an extremely negative judgement at its core. How do you know that individual cases do not represent the whole picture? Therefore, my response is that individual cases represent all of these types of disease, all other cancers, and even all other ever that is in fact not the case at all. .

If the individual cases do not represent the whole picture, then the principle of opening meridians to heal diseases is false. If there are exceptions, it cannot be true that "all illnesses are caused by blocked meridians". Why is there always a difference in the results of PL for the same condition? There are always people who think they are an exception. Because they have individual differences. In fact, the cause of the illness is same as the form of the meridian blockage. People do have very different attitudes towards it. Because people are unpredictable, changeable and have contradictory goals to result in the different results of PL. People have different confidence, doubts and fears about PL, which leads to different times and intensities of Paida, and the amount and type of medication used before and during PL is also very different. For example, one patient was used to heal himself from hypertension, heart disease and kidney disease with PL, which was almost healed. However, later, he had a heart attack and was too lazy to insist on PL. He was frightened by the criticism of Paida in the media, especially when he was admitted to hospital after the HC, and immediately used the medication that he had stopped taking for many years, since he was on the road to deterioration. Later, he tried to PL again. At the time. it was not only difficult to lower his blood pressure and kidney indicators, but the back and leg pain that uses to be resolved with several simple Paida was also ineffective. He sighed that PL was worked for others, while it was not worked for him for the individual differences.

I said, "There is no individual difference, all PL is effective. You are currently using a lot of medications. The negative effects of the medication are also not individualized, which is the reason that your PL is not effective. How can PL be effective when you open the meridians with Paida by 10 points of force and block the meridians with medication by 100 points of force simultaneously? If your Paida is light, how can it be effective if there is no pain or scrapping the bruises out? When it is painful and HC occurs, you are scared and take more medicine and dare not pat on the painful area. How can it be effective?. For example, herbal and western medicines must have negative effects, there are no exceptions. There is different degree to which they work on everyone, it simply means that the mind responds to these negative effects in different ways. For example, you can decide whether to use medicine or not? What kind of medicine to use? How much to use? How to resolve the negative effects? There is no exception to the fact that these medicines have their own effects. The exceptions and the vagaries are caused by the vagaries of the mind.

Moreover, statistically speaking, it is not just individual cases but many cases where PL has been effective for thyroid disease or different kinds of disease. The few cases of thyroid cancer and few people with thyroid cancer who do PL or who have written reports on their cancer and PL. In PL *Clinical Report of Cancer,* you will read about cases of self-healing of different types of cancer.

There are more and less cases of each type depending on the name of disease. For example, there are more cases of lung cancer. These cases are not deliberately chosen by us. However, they appear randomly. Because the multiple cases and the individual cases appear randomly, it proves the higher value of clinical trials, which medicine calls randomized clinical trials. The situation that I have seen is that nobody who has seriously PL with confidence has been ineffective. The more important clinical conclusion is that no matter how different the names of the diseases are, or whether they carry the label of cancer or not, they have the same connotation, i.e. blocked meridians. Therefore, if the meridians are opened, it must be effective.

Looking back in this case, it was certainly not only PL that worked so well, but also the scraping, Primal Point and moxibustion that the patient had used earlier. In particular, the fact that her HC were light indicates that the preliminary treatments were of great help. Please do not forget that these treatments are based on the same principles as PL, they also aim at opening up the meridians. Therefore, it is complementary in terms of opening meridians up. It is fundamentally different from the use of surgery, radiotherapy and drugs that have a greater negative effect. These negative effects are called "negative", rather than "side effect". Because they not only do not open the meridians up, but they can also block them.

In the comprehensive view, it is not surprising that the case was healed for about one month! Does the case represent the whole picture? Certainly, it does! It means that the healing effect of opening up the meridians is universal and absolute without exception! However, the illnesses can only be created and healed by the mind in the final sense, whether a disease can be healed or not can only be determined by the mind. Once you understand that illness is a decision made by the mind for a certain purpose. Healing becomes easier to understand. It may appear that the patient is being assisted by someone or by some means. In fact, assistance is merely a reflection of the choices made. The real doctor is our own mind. It is the mind's choice as to what a person has, what treatment to use and how to use those methods.

The uncertainty of the mind and the contradictory goal of the mind is the root cause of uncertainty and poor healing. Therefore, it can only begin at the source and the mind for real change and healing to take place.

PL can be used as a temporary remedy, or as an "accidental" heal for a medically incurable disease, or it can even be a way to save money or to maintain health for some people. However, it can also unwittingly become a mindfulness technique and lifestyle. If you do PL with your heart as living style, you will find your mind changed, becoming softer and more compassionate, and more willing to share the technique with others. It is not only losing out by sharing, but also gaining more you share. It is something that you cannot achieve by using drugs, tools, doctors, and other external forces. Because you are healing the heart in the name of healing the body.

To further explore the relationship among PL and the heart, mind, HC and lifestyle, please refer to the next case study.

## 1-24 Mystery of HC from the sequelae of hyperthyroidism

**Editor's note: I admired Ms. Deng's calmness in the face of her HC, which is the great self-healing power that regulates the body and mind. Unfortunately, most people are swayed by the wrong culture and habits, who lacks the awareness of self-healing power, so they can be scared by themselves for their own fears to persist and worsen their condition.**

**Ms. Deng comes from Taiwan and works as an executive in a Taiwanese company in Huizhou. During the National Day, she and the chairman of the company, Mr. Chen, came to Shenzhen for a seven-day workshop to provide a comprehensive care for the body. At the end of the workshop, Mr. Chen, the chairman of the company, felt so well physically and mentally that he immediately purchased ten stretching benches to place in his company, so that his**

**staff could also benefit. Ms. Deng and Mr. Chen's good deeds are enabled many more people to benefit from Lajin and Paida. The following is a personal sharing put together by Ms. Deng after she returned home from the course.**

My surname is Deng, I am 45 years old, female, from Taiwan and currently working in a Taiwanese factory in Huizhou.

Stretching is the method of health care that I have insisted on for the longest time. My colleagues laughed at me and said, "Even though you are scraping and shaking your hands at present, you cannot persist on one of these treatments, I suspect that you have brief period of enthusiasm for Paida again." I think that persisting in PL works best for you.

At the beginning of 2009, I started to follow the PL blog and learned about the Lajin method, so that I started to stretch with 2 chairs against the door frame. When I stretch my hands and feet, I know that I am draining the cold. After Lajin, I want to fall asleep at 9:00 pm and sleep deeply at night.

In July 2010 I bought a wooden stretching bench and followed the blog's goal of sticking to it for more than 30 minutes, starting with 10 minutes to 30 minutes for each leg and slowly increasing it. I continued to stretch until one day a colleague asked me: what kind of make-up I was using? How had my face lost its spots and my back straightened up, as it was sore and lame in the pass. A classmate, who I had not seen for a long time, said, "You seem to be different, while I can not speck out your differences." He also spoke with a strong tone of voice that I was convinced of the Lajin method.

Unfortunately, I did not pay attention to the warm spring in April 2011 and caught a cold during the stretching session. Since then, I have been working overtime. All my old health problems have come back to me. Myopia had deepened and my presbyopia had increased, and I was sweating profusely on the hot weather or when I drank hot soup. Thus, I had a strong idea in my mind: I would go to a course to get my body in shape. Since the 11$^{th}$ class was scheduled to start at the right time, I enrolled in the class.

I benefited from the 7-day PL Health Management Course. I enjoyed Paida, Lajin, jogging, meditation, and videos. Every time my palm touched the skin of my face during Paida on the head, I could feel the comforting sensation of Qi, which is slightly numb and comfortable. When I did Lajin on my limbs from back to front, each stroke seems like the pricking of a pin or cutting by a knife. I am grateful to the instructors for helping me to get a lot of deep purple bruises. I knew that I was weak, even I did not realize that my meridians were so badly blocked. When I reached the point of Lajin, the instructor pressed my feet, which was really painful idea.

Jogging: I really enjoyed this class, it was the first time that I jogged barefoot, I was able to breathe in rhythm with my feet, I was sweating all over at the end of class.

On the evening of the fifth day of the course, I started HC (I had hyperthyroidism at 16 years old and had an operation on my abdomen for fibroids at 30 years old), my pulse rate was 100 beats per minute, my whole body was weak, my throat was uncomfortable, and I felt pain in my abdomen. It was hard to sleep all night.

On the morning of the sixth day, the coach encouraged me to run as slowly as possible. I could barely make it to the third or fourth lap when a hot flux spread in my left abdomen and the menstrual pain disappeared. I continued to run despite the discomfort and felt the heat. When I went back to my room and lay down in bed, the heat in my abdomen intensified and spread to my right abdomen and belly button.

Meditation: I was able to focus on my mind with the comfortable music. However, my back was too sore to last until the end.

I learned from Mr. Xiao's video that illness is a result of the "mind's desire" and "all illnesses arise from the mind". At that time, I was a closed-minded, stubborn, and suspicious person, and I really suffered a lot. When the heart shrinks, the tendons shrink; when the tendons shrink, the meridians become blocked, and illnesses come.

By learning PL method, I was able to prevent my body from getting sick. If I want to be healthier, I still must keep up with PL, just as Mr. Xiao said: if you want to get well quickly, just Paida hard; if you want to get well slowly, just Paida gently; if you do not want to get well, please do not start Paida.

It is my wish to keep my body healthy and teach PL to those who need to help.

After the 3 days of fasting, I felt lighter and clearer in my mind; after the course, I started to get in touch with the world, but I do not feel that clarity anymore.

During the process of writing and sharing, I sometimes felt that my mind was short-circuited, so I remembered to pat on the Baihui point as soon as I felt that my mind was short-circuited. My mind became clear, just like an ape ...... It is funny!

I returned to Huizhou on October 6 after an early training session, and then returned to Taipei on October 9, I returned to Huizhou from Taipei until October 19.

HC started on the night of October 5 (pulse: 100 beats per minute, there is general weakness, throat discomfort, accompanied by abdominal menstrual pain; do not sleeping well all night).

On October 6, the weakness was accompanied by a feeling of vomiting, a sore throat and a long gasp before I felt more comfortable. Although I started eating millet porridge, I felt sick in my stomach and vomited some acid. These symptoms are the symptoms of an onset of hyperthyroidism. At the time, I just felt uncomfortable for HC, it was a bit scary in retrospect (the symptoms of HC were worse than my symptoms during hyperthyroidism).

On October 7 to 8, I was still weak with a rapid pulse, ate some soft food. The discomfort in the throat and stomach had been released.

From October 9 to 19, his strength gradually recovered, his heart rate resumed, and most of the black bruises had receded; only the red spot on the third junction of the lower leg remained, there was still a little swelling and pain when I pressed on the lower leg.

On the evening of October 15, I chatted with friends until 3:00 am the next morning.

On the morning of October 16, I squatted down to sort out my belongings and stood up about 10 minutes later, my eyes turned black suddenly, I felt weak, with the fast heartbeat and I would want to vomit. I immediately laid down and rested and did not return to normal until I woke up at 13:00 pm that day; I guessed that it was HC.

On October 20, I started to run in the morning to feel the rising of Yang energy and the lightness of my body. I asked myself to keep on it. Thus, I arranged a health package: 30 minutes of running in the morning at 6:30 am; 108 times of hitting against the wall at 10:00 am; 40 minutes of stretching at 9:30 pm.

I also add a special holiday meal from time to time.

When I returned to Huizhou, I started to run, stretch, and hit the wall in the morning. I was more energetic, I should say more energetic, and I continued to work. I would hope to have more noticeable adjustments after persevering for a period. I would share with you later.

Wish you: Have happiness, satisfactory and health!

--Mrs. Deng, the student from the 11th Shenzhen camp, October 22, 2011

If we look at the effects of healing alone, this case is far less miraculous and dramatic than the healing of the cancer in the previous example. On the contrary, it recounts more of HC that arose during and after PL workshop, there is common status for many people yet: medication, injections and surgery because of previous illnesses, which resulted in the usual fatigue and weakness, back pain, poor immunity, colds and coughs at every turn and others. Therefore, some people call it sub-health. In fact, it is an unhealthy state, rather than a diagnosed name for the disease. It can be diagnosed immediately by PL, it does not use the name of the disease, while the blockage of the meridians to show your condition. The most common blocked meridians in "sub-health" people are the heart, pericardium, and lung meridians. If you had to name them as diseases, they would be heart disease, cardiac disease, and lung disease. These diseases are not as easy to detect as hyperthyroidism or blood pressure, which can be neglected.

The author had experimented with stretching before attending camp, "When my hands and feet got cold when I stretched, I knew that I was draining the cold." It drained the cold from the whole body. First, it drained the cold from the heart and passes through the heart meridian. It was HC. Certainly, "I slept very deeply at night." It was the self-healing effect of HC. Thus, Lajin gradually became a part of her life, increasing the time spent on Lajin each leg from 10 minutes to 30 minutes, she became "clear-headed, refreshed, more energetic...spots were gone, her back was straighter, and her speech was full of energy."

It is pretty good enough. Had her meridians really cleared up? Had all the old illnesses dissolved? Besides, she had only Lajin and did not Paida. Therefore, it was only when she arrived at the workshop and experienced PL that her HC became more comprehensive and deeper. The latent old illnesses were exposed more clearly; it was the deeper diagnosis and healing. "When I did Lajin on my limbs, back and chest, each stroke seems as pricking by pin or cutting by knife. I am grateful to the instructors for helping me to get a lot of deep purple bruises. I knew that I was weak, even I did not realize that my meridians were so badly blocked." The level of pain and scraping showed that her blocked meridians were spread throughout her body and were severely blocked. The pain in her chest and back showed deep blockages in the heart and lung organs and associated meridians, where the deeper HC emerged: "my pulse rate was 100 beats per minute, my whole body was weak, my throat was uncomfortable and I felt pain in my abdomen. It was hard to sleep all night." She just explained that she had hyperthyroidism at 16 years old and an operation for uterine fibroids at 30 years old. You can see how accurate HC are! People often think that they have been healed of their illnesses many years ago. They do not know that the root of the illness has not been removed, i.e. the relevant meridians are still blocked, so that the lesions are still there. HC can turn them out, dissolve them and expel them. It is the clinical manifestation of its treatment and synchronization.

Meanwhile, the effect of Paida on the mind and healing the heart also appears naturally, it is something that each person must understand for himself or herself during Paida, listening and sharing sessions. The human mind and thoughts exist within the mind and operate in accordance with the instructions of the mind. Therefore, the true healing can only begin with a change at the source. The author's analysis of the cause of the illness is honest, as she wrote, "At that time, I was a closed-minded, stubborn and suspicious person. I really suffered a lot. When the heart shrinks, the tendons shrink; when the tendons shrink, the meridians become blocked, and illnesses come." In fact, it is largely true of everyone's sickness process.

HC on the day that she left camp was worth discussing in depth. Because "the symptoms of HC were worse than when I had hyperthyroidism,", "it was a bit scary in retrospect." The symptoms of HC were "the weakness accompanied by a feeling of vomiting, a sore throat and a long gasp before I felt more comfortable. Although I started eating millet porridge, I felt sick in my stomach and vomited acid. These symptoms are the symptoms of an onset of hyperthyroidism that I had forgotten."

The so-called HC means that the lesion existing in the body is first found and flushed out. If no foci exist, there is of course no HC. Therefore, those who have HC should be grateful first that they have found and resolved a disease that is hidden deep inside their bodies. Will the disease be healed automatically if you do not PL? If you really believe it, you are carrying a bomb with you unconsciously when it will explode. When you reviewed it through the lens of Paida, the disease is not terrible. It's just a blockage in the meridians, to put it bluntly. There were the same symptoms of her HC in the following days, which were summarized as blockages in the heart, pericardium, lung, and stomach meridians. The heart and pericardium meridian blockage was manifested as tachycardia and long shortness of breath, the lung meridian blockage was manifested as throat disorders and long shortness of breath, and the stomach meridian blockage was manifested as stomach discomfort and vomiting of acid. PL is the most effective during HC. Because Qi has already flushed the lesions to the surface. When Paida on the elbow fossa and Neiguan acupoint can dissolve all these symptoms simultaneously, including those of stomach discomfort. Unfortunately, she did not PL or forgot how to dissolve HC by Paida when she was suffering from HC.

She chatted on the night of October 15 until the following morning 3:00 am. When she experienced "I squatted down to sort out my belongings and stood up about 10 minutes later, while my eyes turned black suddenly, I felt weak, with the fast heartbeat and I would want to vomit. I immediately laid down and rested and did not return to normal until I woke up at 13:00 pm that day; I guessed that it was HC." Surely, it was HC. If she had done Lajin, Paida on her inner elbow and Neiguan acupoint, it would have dissolved even faster. From the series of HC, it seemed that her heaviest and deepest illness was heart disease, as HC symptoms were always the most obvious ones each time. It showed that the hyperthyroidism that was diagnosed for her in the past was actually heart and lung disease. Because the indicators of hyperthyroidism were the easiest to measure, she was treated as if she had hyperthyroidism all the time. We have discussed several symptoms of post-hyperthyroidism and post-thyroid cancer earlier, all of them were similar, the heart and lung meridians were the most blocked. However, Western medical treatment is symptom-specific, whether it is medication to control the index or surgery to remove the lesion, it is symptomatic without causative, so that the disease may seem to improve, while there are a bunch of sequelae, especially the most obvious panic and fatigue.

However, it is good news that once you know that it is just a blockage in the meridians, it is easy to resolve with PL. The problem is that few people think about PL the whole body to completely resolve the old and new symptoms. After a few full-body Paida sessions, your body and mind are refreshed which comes from clearing out those bombs in your body. You could only feel it by yourself. After a safe landing, it is more important that you integrate PL into your daily life. However, most people do not think so, it would play the dangerous game that I'm talking about, i.e. wait until the illness flares up or gets worse before taking it seriously. The author of this article was able to participate in camp, forced by her illness. As a result, it has made great progress. However, based on her account of HC, she still needs several more full-body Paida sessions to completely dissolve the deep-seated lesions. Once she implemented her health package, it did work. "The whole person was more energetic, it should be said that she has more energy, it was unlike the groggy one before."

However, I noticed that the only thing missing from her package was Paida. Perhaps because she was afraid of pain. Paida was exactly what she needed most for a deep detox. Before she joined the camp, she also only stretched without Paida. Because she did not normally pat, Paida seems as pricking by pin or cutting by knife at the camp. She also never used the pat during many HC sessions. Whether the decision not to pat was caused by fear, doubt, or other reasons, it was clearly a decision of the mind. It can also be said that it is exactly HC of heart disease.

# Chapter 3 Clinical discussion of goiter, nodule, tumor and cyst

The diagnosis of hyperthyroidism, hypothyroidism, thyroiditis and thyroid cancer must be confirmed by examination of the relevant biological indicators, whereas a mass in the thyroid gland is obvious on visual inspection. Although the mass refers to the different names in different cases, such as enlargement, nodule, tumor, cyst and others. Two categories also intersect with each other and are slightly categorized only for ease of discussion and reference. Although thyroid disorders are divided into so many different names by Western medicine, they are essentially the same in PL method, all of them were caused by the multiple blockages of heart, lung and large intestine meridians. Therefore, there are no different healing methods. It may sound oversimplified; it is exactly clinical verification.

## 2-1 Goiter cyst was healed by Paida of two elbows for 10 minutes

I once did Paida a friend down 10 minutes in total, I patted down her goitre, which was the size of a half egg in the past.

At the end of 2018, my friend told me about a thyroid cyst and after seeing several major hospitals and several specialists, she was advised to have it surgically removed to prevent it from becoming lesions.

Once, we were having dinner together and I saw that she was fatter than usual at that time, I asked her after dinner, "How is your blood pressure these days?" She said, "It's a bit high". At that time, I was not afraid of anything and asked her if I help her to do Paida on the back. She agreed. I patted her elbows with a lot of bruises in just 10 minutes.

The next day she called me to tell me that I had crippled her hands and that she could not move them. I immediately thought of HC and I asked her if you had ever had any injuries to your hands in the past. She said she had an accident in the past and her hand was hit. I said it did not matter; it would be healed in a few days.

I wanted to pat her again, there was no time, she went abroad. Three months later, when I saw her again, the thyroid cyst had disappeared cleanly without any trace.

I asked her if she had taken any medication, any injections, or other treatments in the intervening months. She said nothing.

She had been injured in the past and her meridians were blocked, so the toxins in her body could not be expelled and piled up in her thyroid gland, to form a thyroid cyst. A lot of bruises came out for 10 minutes of Paida, which cleared up the blockages in the meridians. The toxins in the thyroid gland slowly came out, and the thyroid cyst cleared up on its own.

--Huaimin, 2021.8.31

I said that hypertension was a symptom of heart disease that it is caused by blockages in the heart meridian and pericardium meridian. Therefore, the pat for hypertension is the same method as for heart disease, Paida of the elbow fossa can lower hypertension. Of course, if the blood pressure is low, Paida of the elbow fossa will raise it. You will see a large number of cases in PL *Clinical Report for Heart Disease* and PL *Clinical Report for High/Low Blood Pressure*. Nowadays, there are many diseases as hyperthyroidism, hypothyroidism and goitre, which are also caused by blockages in the heart, pericardium and lung meridians. It can also be resolved by Paida on the elbow. This case is a clinical demonstration.

It was originally intended to treat hypertension, while the thyroid cyst was resolved, which seems to be a misnomer. It looks like the right thing to do. Because the cause of hypertension and thyroid is blockage of the heart, pericardium, and lung meridians. The Paida of two elbows opened these three meridians together. It is like shooting three hawks with one arrow. In addition to two diseases, the trauma suffered on the hands in the past was also resolved in a HC. The bruises coming out and the inability to move her hands were HC.

## 2-2 Paida the thumb and fissure acupoint for two hours, thyroid nodules were healed

I went to hospital in May this year for a routine physical examination. A thyroid nodule was found on my right side. The outpatient clinic for further treatment was recommended by the doctor. However, I have been putting it off.

Last night after 9:00 pm, my right thumb (palm side) tingled a bit from time to time, I could feel the kind of pain from blocked meridians, so that I did Paida my thumb. After nearly an hour, the rest of the thumb did not hurt as much, except for Yuji acupoint, which was still particularly painful and swollen.

After Paida for half hour, the pain was still as painful and swollen as it had been at the Yuji acupoint. I knew in my heart that "Blockage accompanies to pain", so I did Paida with all my strength for two or three times, it was so painful.

After three times of Paida, the pain point ran to the surface of the skin, the big blue and purple silt block came out simultaneously, there was a little pain at the neck, and then touched the nodule with my hand. It was found that the nodule was gone and flat, it was nearly 11:00 pm, I was sleepy and went to bed.

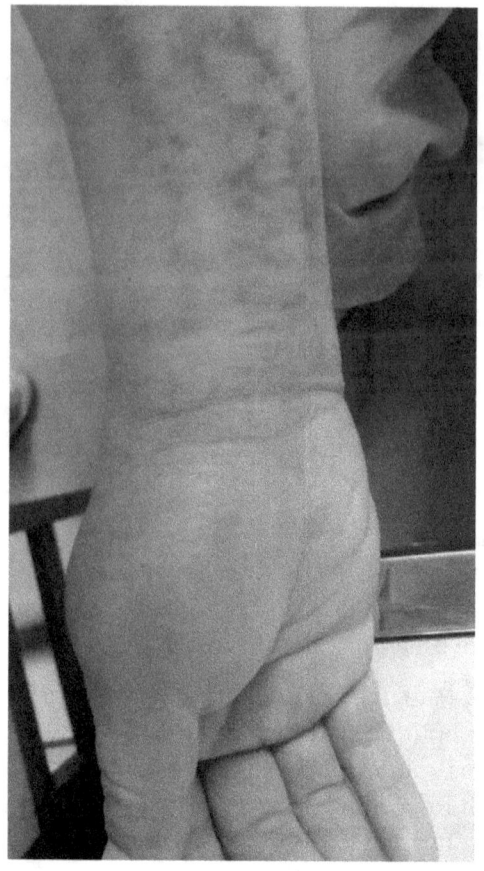

I woke up early this morning and looked in the mirror and the left and right sides of my neck became the same, the knot on the right side of the node was gone, just a little sore and a little red at the skin. Oh my God. I can not believe that it is true, the nodules just disappeared so easily.

I searched for the function of the Yuji acupoint in Baidu ...... It was the right remedy. I would share it to people with the same condition, thyroid nodules have a chance of becoming cancerous, which is not a disease to treat easily. Is the interthyroidal point the original point for thyroid nodules? Why else would it be so immediately obvious? I am purely a blind cat meeting a dead mouse, lucky and happy. I am grateful to PL, as well as the advocates of PL!

--A netizen, 2021-06-15

The author pats the inner thumb and the Yuji acupoint, both of which belong to the lung meridian. The lung travels up through the diaphragm via the middle epiglottis, connecting the lungs, through the trachea and throat, across the armpit, then through the inner elbow and Yuji acupoint, and end at the tip of the thumb. The meridian runs through the throat where the thyroid gland is located, so she has opened up a blockage in the meridian where the thyroid gland is located by Paida of the lung meridian. The area between the fissure and the pericardium meridian is almost connected. When she did Lajin the fissure she must have done Lajin to the pericardium meridian as well. Paida differs from acupuncture for which the stimulation area is larger and more intense in Paida.

Although the two hours were spent simply patting on the meridian, a total of four HC came out: 1) Extra pain in the thumb when did Lajin; 2) Pain, swelling and swelling at the Yuji acupoint; 3) A large, bruised blood packet on the surface of the piriformis; and 4) Pain at the neck, where HC of the thyroid nodule. Four sites of HC were extremely precise, which were diagnosed as blocked meridians and sites, and the degree of blockage was revealed. Meanwhile, the foci of disease were resolved, among which the nodules were also kind of foci of disease.

## 2-3 The size of thyroid nodule became negligible after two times of Paida

I had a thyroid nodule that the I was required to be hospitalized for before Paida, I declined to be hospitalized and take the medication. The journey of testing the size of the nodules in my neck began every 3 months.

Then I came across PL, which led to a great improvement in my scapulohumeral periarthritis by the prone Lajin method at the first time. The limb aches and pains were relieved by Paida. I had a sudden thought: PL can expel waste from the body, and the nodules in the neck were also waste from the thyroid gland, so they should be expelled from the body.

Therefore, I started PL by myself...I would have the pain of Paida, rather than the pain of surgery.

In addition to Paida of the general area, Paida of neck was also conducted directly for 2 times, each time four hours, with two interval weeks, lasting for a total of one month. An ultrasound at week 5 showed that the size of the nodules in the neck was negligible!

The specific approach was shown as below:

1. Paida on the general area.
2. Lie flat on your back and adopt a recumbent position for the neck Lajin method.
3. Start Paida on the upper edge of the right pectoralis major muscle with the palm of your left hand for 5 minutes, gradually do Paida upwards on the right side of the clavicle and neck to the right side of the jaw.
4. Start Paida gradually and forcefully (the neck is very sensitive to pain) so that Paida of area is slowly adapted to the pain.
5. Start Paida the left pectoralis major with the right hand (as in 3.4).
6. After the neck has adapted to the pain in the front and back, switch to Paida board again and continue to Paida for four hours. Thus, Paida of the neck could be comprehensive, thorough, and effective.
7. Keep the neck warm after Paida.

After two weeks, when the bruises in the neck have basically disappeared, start Paida of neck again ......

My humble opinion: Paida yourself and stick to the pain for best results. The pain of Paida on the neck is not comparable to the pain of neck surgery. Insist on PL for your own health.

I have a low level of education with poor expressions, it is used for reference only. Please understand! Thank you, PL! Thank you, my husband!

My nodules have become smaller through twice Paida of neck ...... My confidence of my health is stronger!

-- Ms. Wei from Qingdao, June 30, 2018

It is a classic case of an illness being treated by heart. The doctor had originally admitted her to hospital, she refused. Her mind decided as below, "I would have the pain of Paida, rather than the pain of surgery." There is the truth that surgery is more damaging. Because the surgery destroys the meridians and causes permanent damage. PL is easy, it is not easy for making up your mind to do this decision. Most people do not believe in PL.

Her clinical account of PL has been described in detail. I just need to summarize it from a meridian perspective. Firstly, she did Lajin on the general area, which already did Lajin on the heart, lung and large intestine meridians associated with the thyroid once. She focused on Paida the neck circle and the area around the collarbone. As the neck is where the three Yin Meridians and three Yang Meridians converge in the hands, the clavicle is where the three Yin meridians converge, namely the heart, lung and pericardium meridians. She has the most pain when she pats the neck, which is HC, which indicated that that is where the blockage is greatest. In short, any illness of the thyroid gland is the result on a blockage of these 6 meridians.

She mentioned that she had improved her scapulohumeral periarthritis with lying stretches, which has been beneficial in self-healing thyroid disease. Because the shoulder is also where the 6 meridians of the hands centering together, the heart, pericardium and lung meridians are located on the front side, and the large intestine, small intestine and Tri-jiao meridians are located on the middle and back side.

## 2-4 How to Paida on the breast tumor and thyroid tumor?

I have been PL for two years without interruption and have benefited a lot from it. Even my rheumatoid arthritis, which cannot be healed by Chinese and Western medicine, has been restored to the normal status by PL. During the period, I also often help my family and friends to pat, so I Paida with my hands also use a Paida tool as it is more handy, brilliant, and the doubly effective. (Every potter praises his pot)

In the beginning, I patted myself with two hands. After a period, the bruises did not come out much. I knew that the root of disease had not yet been removed. Besides, Paida of parts, such as the roots of the thighs, back, buttocks, fingers, toes, collarbone and others areas fell short and the Paida tool became very effective in bringing out sha.

Then I bought a variety of Paida boards in the different sizes, domestic and foreign, cheap and expensive, soft and hard. However, the results were not too satisfactory until I bought a silicone Paida board, which is food-grade silicone and can come into direct contact with the skin. I love that I even take it all the time when I travel. (I seem to be talking about a couple of lovers).

In fact, Paida of two hands can combine with a good Paida board for better effectiveness. How to pat?

Firstly, it shall be mentioned that: the board with bigger particles shall be used first, for it can pat deep enough. (The side with smaller particles will be shallower). Secondly, the front end of the Paida board with a lot of elasticity shall be used to avoid pain and produce more bruises. (the middle of the Paida board will be harder and more painful). Thirdly, the whole body can be patted with Paida board (except for the eyes). Many people have asked me: can I pat on the bones or among the bones, as well as the head, face, neck and muscles? The answer is: all of them!

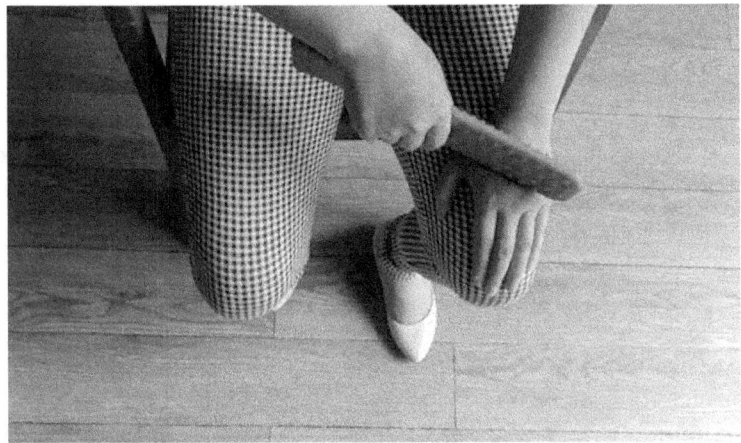

If you use the sideways of board for chopping, with the method of chopping as kitchen knife, the strength is greater, more concentrated and deeper. Sometimes, the bruises come out from the bottom only the day after the beat, its power should not be underestimated. However, the side chopping method requires patience and a longer time. (Because the side area of Paida board is thin)

I kept one month of closed-door PL myself for the severe condition, with a total of 10 hours of PL everyday, so that my rheumatoid arthritis was self-healed completely.

My father's trigger fingers were chopped with the sideways of Paida board, 360 degrees of each section was patted repeatedly. When my mother had an early tumor in her breast, the doctor asked her to have tissue drawn for tests. However, she refused in case the tissue spread. Therefore, I patted the tumor for my mother with the front end of Paida board and then constantly chopped the tumor with the side of board, as chopping a meatloaf. After several times of chopping, the tumor disappeared completely.

There was also my mother's thyroid tumors, which added up to more than a dozen on two sides, which disappeared without a trace by Paida in the way. There are many more effective cases, so I will share them another time to avoid lengthiness.

In some cases, I would pat the patient's left and right sides simultaneously as the volunteer. However, my PL was effective. There were also cases where I would pat the patient with different paddles simultaneously, while my PL was still effective. There were certain illnesses that was slow to recover. Once the Paida board is used, recovery can be rapid by the method. Given the many experiences with Paida by self, other PL and feedback from friends, the method recommended above has proven to be superior.

Please do not misunderstand me for making an advertising campaign. There are too many people have benefited from my recommendations. In order to introduce its benefits for more people, I would share my own experiences by the online platform. Of course, PL with hand, PL with Paida board, PL with side chopping shall aim at one purpose: get rid of illnesses and improve health!

--Eva, Hong Kong, 2014-4-3

Eva is already a legend in the history of PL. Her record of Paida for a month and 10 hours a day has be broken yet. The case is a report of PL on her mother to resolve an early tumor. Based on her own and her mother's full confidence in PL, she refused to take a biopsy for tissue chemistry. "I patted the tumor for my mother with the front end of Paida board and then constantly chopped the tumor with the side of board, as chopping a meatloaf. After several times of chopping, the tumor disappeared completely."

Mammary tumors, fibroids and thyroid tumors often co-exist and the several cases were seen. Her mother's thyroid tumor, "There was also my mother's thyroid tumor, which added up to more than a dozen on two sides, which disappeared without a trace by Paida in the way." Looking at the clinical process, it is as simple as the first case discussed in this chapter, which is to pat directly on the affected area. For those who are afraid of pain or have complex conditions, the generic area and surrounding areas can be patted first, before concentrating on the affected area. This decision is too difficult to make for many people. In this case, the author's mother and father had healed themselves from a variety of difficult illnesses by PL, it is only natural to heal themselves from a variety of tumors by PL. The mind determines the fate of the body.

The author has mentioned many times in other case studies that she usually spends half an hour for PL on each part. Only places are changed after she has patted thoroughly. It is her usual style of Paida and one of the secrets of her success.

## 2-5 Thyroid and gynecological problems were all improved at physical examination after PL

Hello, everyone! I am 53 years old and have many problems. I felt dizzy everyday and can not walk steadily. In 2012, I had a herniated disc in my lower back. I also had constant pain in my sciatic bone, the knee and lumbar ischia is degenerative diseases. I felt very tired and exhausted going up the stairs. The breast was tested as BI-RADS category 4a on the left side and category 3 on the right side since 2016.

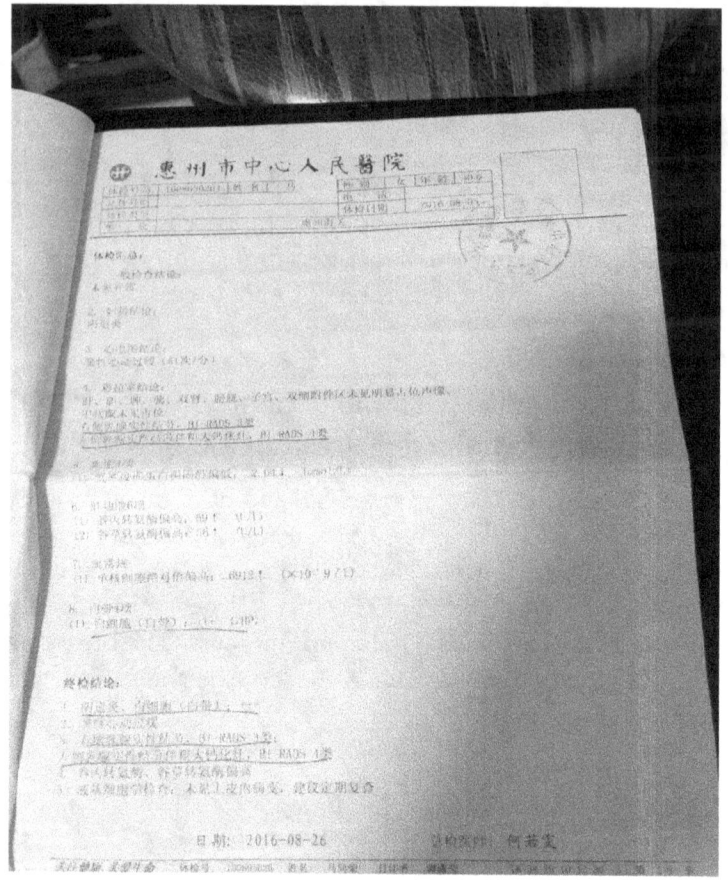

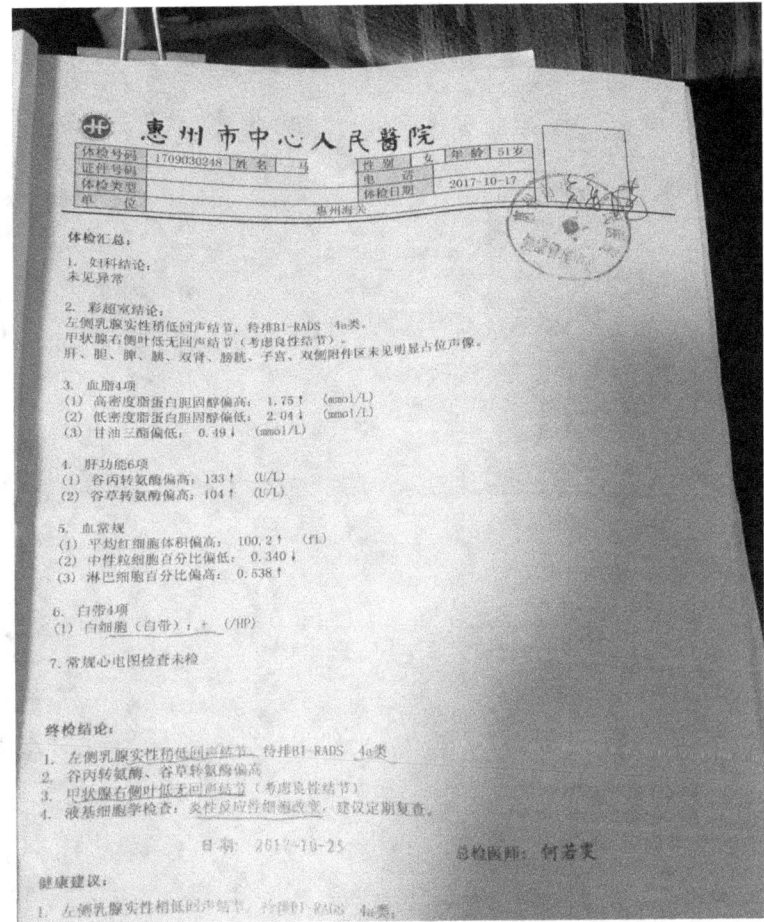

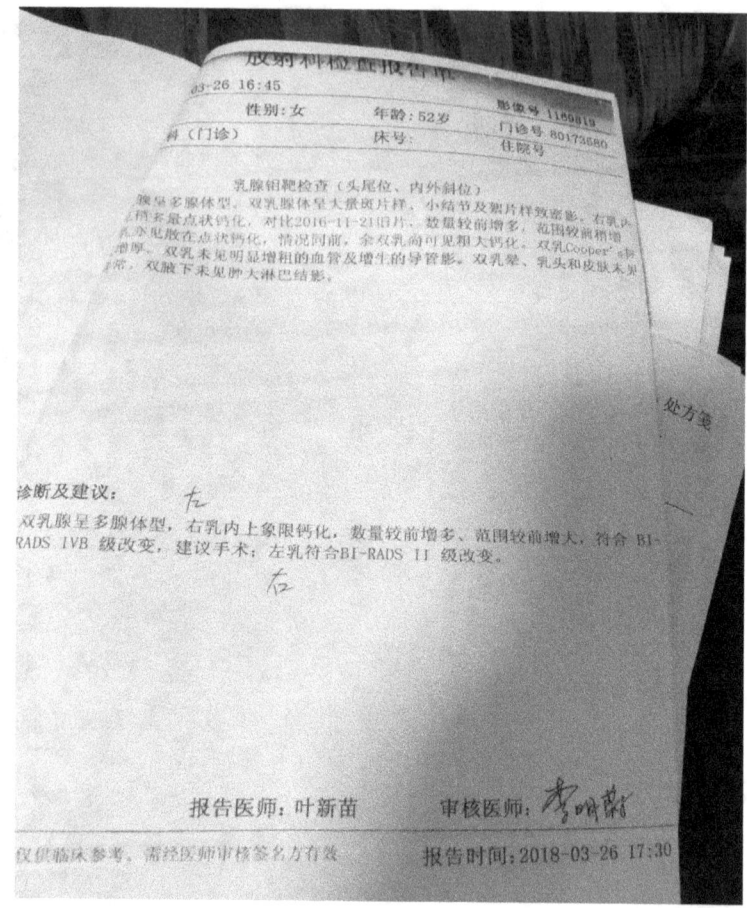

    I had surgery to remove fibroids on the left side of the breast in April this year. Inflammatory problems in gynecology have always been there. After I was massaged by a folk doctor in 2016, legs and feet had been swollen until now and the swelling has not gone yet.

    I started PL on June 20, 2018. Starting from the generic area, when I patted until black bruises came out at the beginning, I thought that the blood vessels were broken, I immediately stopped not daring to pat again. Later, through reading books, reading others' exchanges in the group, and the links posted by teachers in the group, I slowly became unafraid.

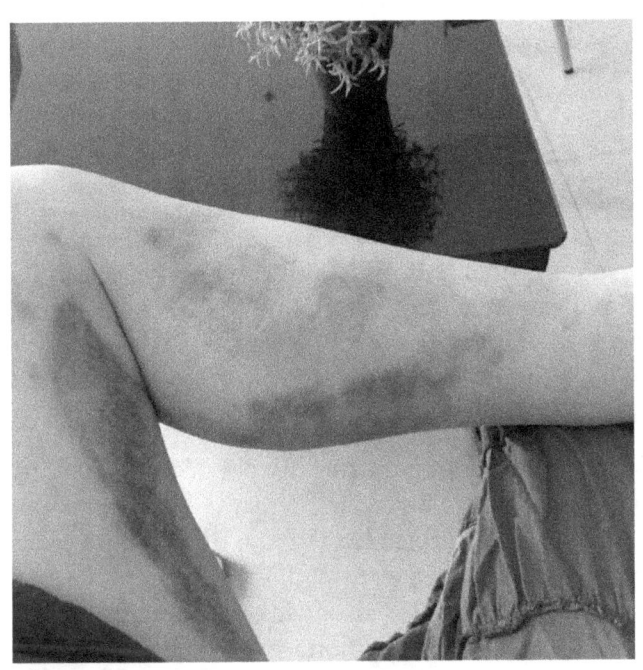
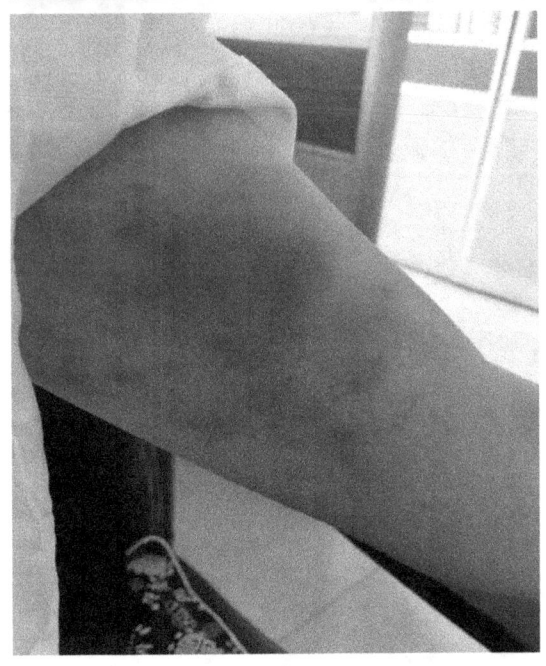

After that, I kept PL everyday, I did more Paida in my spare time, while I did less PL when I did not have enough time. Sometimes, I just stood on the stretching board when I did not have time. I had a serious problem with my body, as I swelled up when I did it, especially in my lower body, and I would swell up for a few weeks.

After a month, I felt that my health condition had not improved significantly, and my symptoms had worsened. I was envious of others who could see immediate results with a single pat, so I wondered why it was so difficult for me to make a difference.

Ms. Zhang Yumei kept encouraging me, said that HC can take a long time to get through, and told me that I should read more books to learn about the principles of PL and read more about other people's cases to increase my confidence; the teacher Mo Fei and Amethyst in the group was also guiding me everyday. I just insisted on PL, my physical condition was so bad, it can be solved for a while, I did not expect to achieve any improvement soon. I just did PL everyday as usual.

On September 11, I conducted the physical examination, and the results came back on September 18, I found several changes that I did not expect:

## 我的体检报告

报告导读　总检报告　医师建议　指标明细

1. 一般检查结论：
未见异常

2. 耳鼻喉科结论：
咽部:咽炎

3. 妇科结论：
未见异常

4. 心电图结论：
窦性心动过缓（56次/分）

5. 彩超室结论：
甲状腺未见明显占位性病变
双侧乳腺未见明显占位性病变：符合BI-RADS 1类。
肝、胆、脾、胰、双肾、膀胱、子宫及双侧附件区未见占位

6. 血脂4项
(1) 高密度脂蛋白胆固醇偏高： 1.64↑ (mmol/L)

7. 肾功3项
(1) 尿素测定偏低： 2.3↓ (mmol/L)

8. 血常规
(1) 中性粒细胞百分比偏低： 0.399↓
(2) 淋巴细胞百分比偏高： 0.509↑
(3) 中性粒细胞绝对值偏低：1.6758↓ ($\times 10^9$/L)

9. 尿常规＋沉渣定量（仪器法）
(1) 潜血：2.0-5.0(+2) (mg/L)

1. 咽炎
2. 窦性心动过缓
3. 双侧乳腺未见明显占位性病变
4. 尿潜血阳性
5. 液基细胞学检查：未见上皮内病变或恶性病变（NILM）

医师建议

总检医生：何若雯　　总检日期：2018-08-31

1. 咽炎：
请到耳鼻喉科就诊咨询。

2. 窦性心动过缓：
窦性心动过缓常见于健康的年轻人、运动员、老年人以及某些疾病或服用某些药物的人。无症状的窦性心动过缓通常不需治疗，如显著持久的窦性心动过缓（心率＜50次/分），造成心排血量不足伴有头晕，乏力等症状的，请到心内科进一步诊治。

3. 双侧乳腺未见明显占位性病变：
体检结果正常，请一年后复查。

1. My physical examination indicated with an enlarged thyroid gland last year, it is normal in this year.
2. In previous years, there was inflammation of the cervix with three plus. Even it was a few degrees of cervical erosion in the past, the cervix is smooth this year.
3. From 2016, BI-RADS category 4 in the left breast, category 3 lesions in the right breast. In April this year, the left side of breast fibroids were removed by surgery. In September this year, the physical examination indicated

that the bilateral breast no obvious occupying lesions: it was consistent with BI-RADS category 1.
4. My height was 164.5-165 cm at physical examination in previous years. However, I am measured as 166 cm in this year.

I can not even believe it that I have only been PL for less than 3 months, my gynecological problems are almost resolved.

It is so strange. I even do not feel these improvements myself. While, the indicators had been changed, and the original change has happened unconsciously.

My worst problems are still lumbar, sciatic and knee pain, as well as swollen legs and feet. While it can be healed that I can manage on my own given some time.

After reviewing the results of my physical examination, Ms. Zhang Yumei told me, "You know when you are uncomfortable, do not over worry about the indicators in the hospital, just PL when you are not feeling well! Paida shall be taken as your daily health care!" Yes, PL is not accomplished at one stroke, and it is not efficacious forever. PL is a daily health care routine that does not cost money and requires less trip to hospital and less medication.

I am grateful to our teachers for passing on the simplest and most practical method of self-healing to the world, so that ordinary people can achieve self-healing and health through their own practice. I am also grateful to the volunteer teachers for their selfless dedication. I wish that there be less suffering, less sickness and less pain in the world. Everyone will be happy and healthy!

--Mrs Ma, from Huizhou, Guangdong, 2018-9-19

This case is characterized by a complex condition under a simple PL, a comprehensive healing process with a sceptical mentality.

In addition to the abnormalities of the various indicators examined in the hospital, her illness obviously felt five or six kinds of pain from head to toe. If more than a dozen diseases are treated with medicine, how many kinds of drugs do you get? Moreover, drugs are generally aimed at symptoms and the cause is unknown. Thus, we must discuss the significance of medical diagnosis. There are many detailed and accurate indicators for diagnosing symptoms. However, does this help to treat the disease? It just like analysis of darkness thoroughly, does analysis of darkness bring light? Why can many people not be healing or their diseases even be aggravated in the hospital for many years? Because the advantage of the hospital only can check the disease, its disadvantage is that the cause cannot be detected, for which it is difficult to heal the disease.

Besides, let's talk about the simplicity of PL. The ordinary people can learn it in a few minutes, it is easy to find the common parts on the limbs. She was able to improve her goitre and many gynecological conditions in three months by the simple method. Why can a simple method improve multiple diseases simultaneously? Because the cause of each disease is simply a blockage of the meridians. For example, thyroid and breast diseases are caused by blockages in the heart, lung and pericardium meridians on the arms and the large intestine, small intestine and Tri-jiao meridians, while uterine diseases are mostly caused by blockages in the liver, spleen and kidney meridians on the feet. Thus, all these diseases can be naturally improved by Paida of limbs.

Why is still doubt in her mind? Because she currently does not understand HC. Therefore, she was sceptical and fearful. "Whenever I was patting, I got swollen, especially in my lower body... the symptoms even become worse. I am depressing why it is so hard for me to have an improvement." Although her perceptions had been corrected through reading and studying the principles and asking for advice in the group, she still lacked in-depth experience. The medical report only gave her an improvement in her indicators, the pain that made her feel most afflicted had not improved yet. On the flip side, the pain was a clear signpost to guide her to PL. If she had really taken the time and effort to pat the painful areas and her whole body properly, the pain would be gone, she would also have better indicators on her re-examination.

This test report had given her more confidence. Her confidence was shown on her enforcement strength. The efficient way was attending a workshop. The next best thing was finding someone to pat each other's whole body. Of course, you can also do PL yourself. However, greater confidence and determination shall be required. For example, Eva locked herself in a room for a month without seeing anyone and PL for 10 hours a day, her whole body can be self-healed for over 20 diseases. If you have the patience, you can also take your time with PL as part of your health care routine. However, the author had severe back pain, sciatica, knee pain and swelling of both legs and feet, rather than health care. The choice of PL can only be decided by your own mind.

## 2-6 Thyroid surgery was canceled by 5 days of Paida

Hello, everyone! My husband had difficulty swallowing at breakfast on the 7th day of the first month, and a mirror revealed that the enlarged thyroid gland, which was found last year, had grown much larger. The ultrasound showed that it was 1 cm larger than when it was discovered 8 months ago, which caused pressure on the trachea and esophagus, and the doctor said that surgery was required.

I was the beneficiary of PL and told my husband that the growth was actually a warning from his body that the blockage was extreme and that if he just cut the bag without clearing the meridians, it would still grow afterwards.

At first, the pouch and the inner side of the upper arm was patted in order. Every inch of skin patted was lumpy as the toad's skin. After Paida for two nights, an hour each night, he was not willing to do Lajin intermittently. He took two slices of ginger each morning.

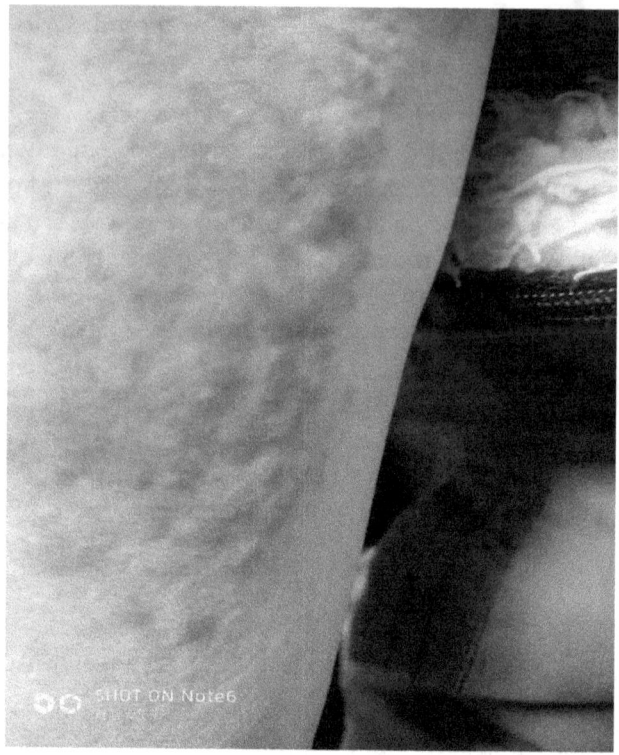

On the morning of the third day, he was excited to say that he felt much better, his breathing was smoother, there was no more pressure in his swallowing. Moreover, the acid reflux that used to occur whenever he ate sweet potatoes, glutinous, rice and other food had disappeared. I had not heard any more thunderous snoring for a few nights.

It's been only 5 days since I took the shots today. It is amazed to see the amazing results. He is now more active about it, he stands on the stretching board at home in his spare time. At night, he takes his coat off and is actively asking to Paida. The reduction in size of the lump is not obvious. Since the pressure is gone, it must be getting smaller and continues to PL!

-- Mrs. Chen, February 22, 2019

The medical examination was accurate. While the examination and the desired surgery aim at a medical condition, the blockage of the meridians causes goitre, which medicine does not even have a concept yet. The author's analysis was simple: "If you just cut the lesions without unblocking the meridians, it will still grow if you cut it. He was advised to PL and then start PL for him at night."

In addition to the lesion, she patted the inner side of the upper arm, which produced a "toad-skin and lumpy" bruise. The areas of bruises were located on the heart, pericardium and lung meridians." On the morning of the third day, he was excited that he felt better, and he could breath better, without the sense of pressure during swallowing. He had acid reflux when he ate sweet potatoes and glutinous rice in the past, it was gone now." It meant that the growth of the mass was only the symptom of appearance, and the blockage of the heart and lung meridians had already caused the breathing, swallowing and acid reflux symptoms. "I do not hear the thunderous grunts anymore," which further indicated that his heart and lungs had long been sick, only the indicators were not easily measured, as the goitre. In short, the heart and lung disease of patient has really been healed or improved. Goiter was just the symptom of two diseases. Was it worth to exempt an operation after 5 times of Paida? However, she clearly had many other meridians throughout her body where were not working and could not be expected to dissolve them with several Paida of arms. PL was still the dangerous games, as it was forced by the aggravating illness. Only when more blocked meridians are opened up and the daily PL habit is developed for the whole body, can it be regarded as entering a safe and happy game.

## 2-7 My familial thyroid nodules are gone

Hi everyone, this is Wind. Coach Liu Ying just asked me to share, I do not know that how to start it suddenly.

As for my thyroid nodules, which run in my family and develop every few years. The symptoms would appear as: a large lump evident on the left side, panic attacks, insomnia, eat heavily and being hungry all the time.

I took Chinese herbal medicine for a year and a half when I had an attack in 2017. I had suffered from another attack in 2020. At the end of the year, I started to learn PL, buy the Self-Healing Method textbook. Then, I attend a small resonance class with Coach Liu Ying, the basic class, a manipulation class and a carpet class. By following the teacher along the way and practically Paida every palm, many minor indisposition and the thyroid nodules were gone. I am grateful to my teacher and PL.

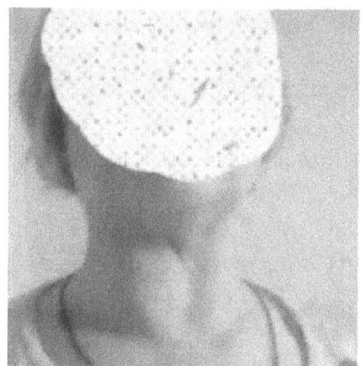 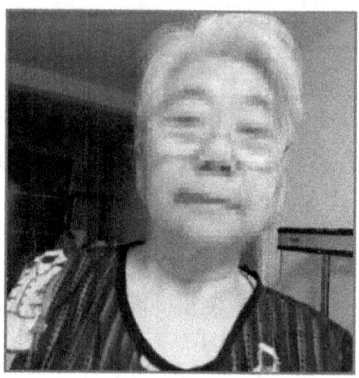

Before and after pictures of PL for thyroid nodules

Apart from attending classes, I mostly followed the 15 video lessons on thyroid nodule problems in the Fangyuan Health app, except for the tenth lesson where the head and face were filmed everyday, and one lesson was taken everyday for other lessons. In principle, I followed the course equipped with stretching, which I changed myself to pulling the cervical spine before waking up in the morning, patting the head and face, standing on the stretching bench after meals, following the course in the morning and patting for one lesson, doing lying Lajin in the afternoon and Y-shape Lajin before sleeping.

-- Feng, 2022.6.21

There are 5 symptoms listed by the author: thyroid nodules, heartburn, insomnia, eating heavily and being hungry all the time. Nodules are only one of them and get attention for the obvious appearance. The most important of these diseases is heart disease. All five symptoms are complications of heart disease, even easy hunger. The blockage of the heart and pericardium meridians can also lead to blockage of the lung, large intestine, small intestine, and stomach meridians, which caused an imbalance in the entire digestive tract. It is called inflammation caused by dysbiosis in western medicine, also known as "leaky gut syndrome". It is difficult for nutrients to be absorbed, so that one is always hungry. In other words, any blockage in the heart meridian will generally lead to different degrees of blockage in all meridians of the body, which can result in a variety of complications.

She attended three kinds of network camps until the carpet class, which showed that she did Lajin on her whole body. Thus, it worked well. The whole body of PL shall be conducted in order to completely dissolve the diseases.

## 2-8 My thyroid gland became smaller after Paida

Hello, everyone. Today, I would like to share my PL process with you. I come from Zhenjiang, Jiangsu Province. I am 66 years old. I believe that I have always had no health problems and I attended the Shanghai PL offline class in 2017.

My health is generally okay, without major problems, hypertension, diabetes and others. I rarely catch a cold in general. However, I like to take care of my health, and I actively learn anything that is good for my body.

I have been studying PL for several years. However, I never did Paida seriously, I just did Paida in my spare time.

I have benefited myself from PL and promote the method to my relatives and friends.

For example, I met a relative in Chongqing who had been in a car accident more than 30 years ago. Two legs swung back and forth like a duck when she walked. At that time, I patted her legs, and it took about four or five hours on the first day. The next day after Paida, she said that her thyroid gland felt smaller. It was true. I did not realize that her thyroid gland became smaller by Paida of her legs inadvertently, it has been getting smaller everyday.

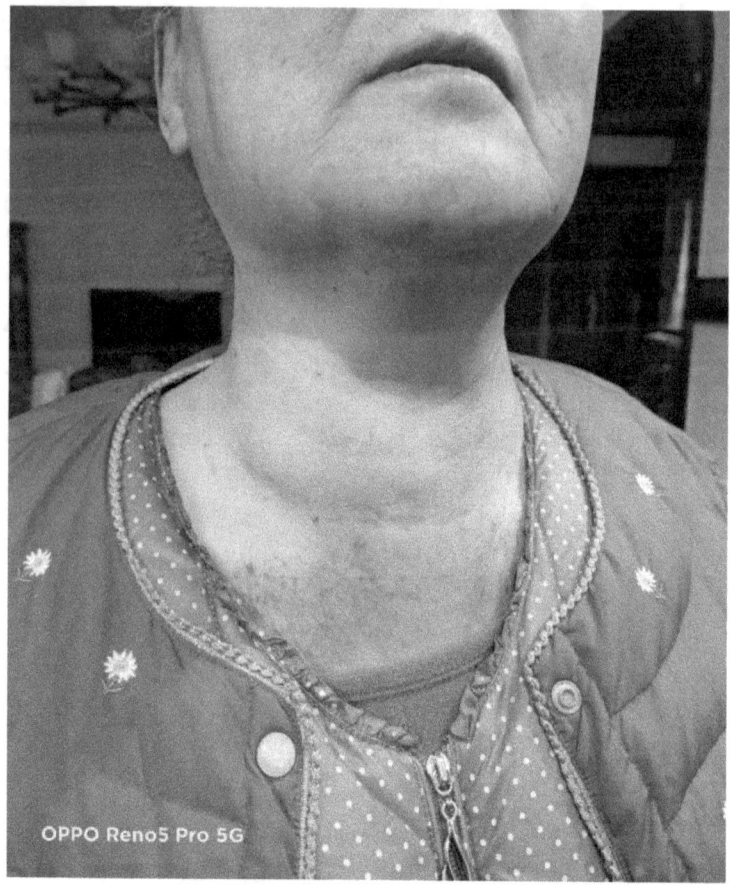

It is her neck after the photo, the swelling on the right side of her neck has gone.

She had surgery on her left neck and the hospital told her to do it on her right neck , she did not do the surgery. After I helped patting on her leg this time, the right side of her neck was getting smaller and she was happy that Paida of her leg had improved her thyroid. In fact, I do not know where the thyroid gland is blocked, it was an unintentional effect of Paida.

Let's talk about my situation of Paida. I had a sore throat two days for some reason. I attended to Paida of overall body class. After I followed the class for two days, my throat stopped hurting and I stopped coughing. On the fourth day, after Paida of arm, I patted my fingers. Since my fingers were not patted in place, I added an afternoon to pat my thumb and index finger. After Paida, a lot of bruises came out. My hands were swollen. All bruises disappeared at the next day.

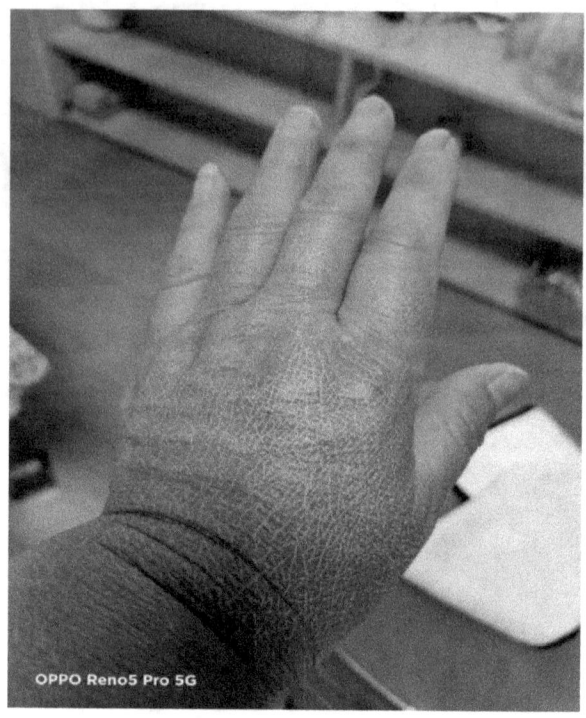

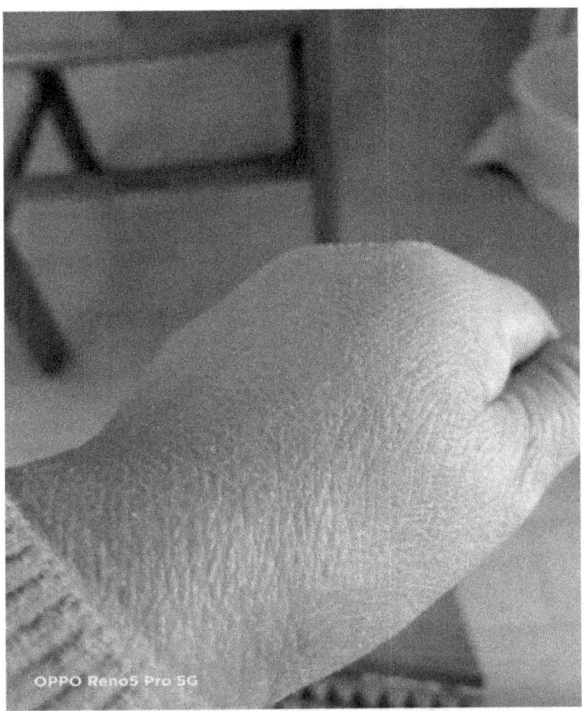

The day before Paida All bruises on the whole hand were gone, it was not swollen anymore the next day.

I had also noticed a reaction in the past few days: I always spit a lot of clear phlegm, and I also run a lot of snot. I guessed that should be HC, where the lesions had been expelled out by Paida. My throat and lungs were particularly relaxed and comfortable in the past two days.

I would like to share a bit more about the benefit obtained from Paida of my legs today. After I did Paida my legs today, I could go up and down the stairs easily and my legs did not feel tired at all. When I went upstairs, I usually felt a tendon twisting and hurting. However, I did not have this feeling today.

In fact, it was very painful during Paida on my leg today, I thought about what my teacher said: the more painful it is, the more I shall pat. The pain was aggravated when I patted it hard. I insisted on it even though it hurt, so the bruises came out well today.

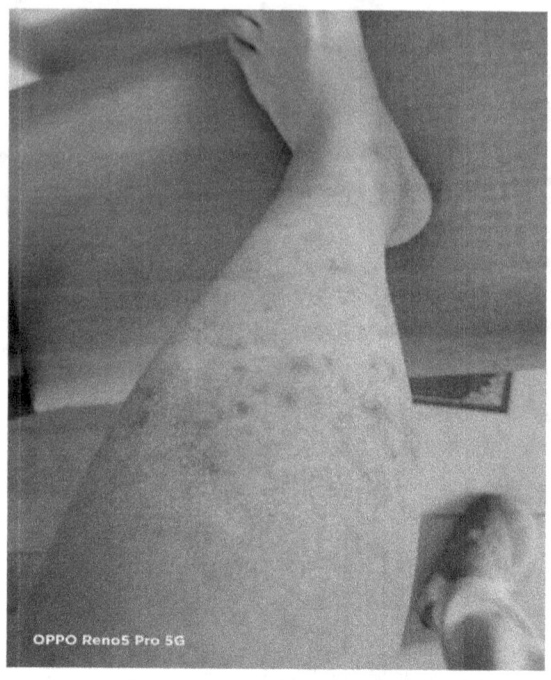

I'm not usually talkative. Please understand if I do not speak well. I had finished my sharing. Thank you!

-- Green Water and Mountain, 2022.4.18

The correct action done by the author seems to be a misrepresentation, which is actually playing the same tune on different instruments. It inadvertently proves the holographic character of meridian healing, whereby each meridian contains information about the entire meridian network. Each body part contains information about the organs and the whole body. *The Invisible Rainbow* written by Zhang Changlin, scientists have proved the truth by the special experiments. In my article "Why PL can self-heal from COVID-2019 pneumonia?" I quoted the results of the experiments from her book.

"From a measurement point of view, every point of the body is a micro meridian point. This idea is further supported by the technique of electrical measurement of meridian points. Since it is assumed that every point of the whole body is a micro-meridian point, a random measurement is used, that is, a blind measurement with the eyes closed. Because every point in the body is an acupoint according to holographic thinking, no matter how it is measured blindly, it is always measured at a particular micro-meridian point. There is no way to get it wrong. Because it is holographic. Interestingly, the scientists' speculations were confirmed by the results of the experiment. The probability distribution curves of the conductance data are similar regardless of which area of the body is measured." (*The Invisible Rainbow* P95-96)

Why are effective for treating diseases with ear acupuncture and nasal acupuncture by acupuncturists? Because the small area of ear and nose had many acupuncture points that reflect all the organs of the body. The diagnosis and pointing of the sole of the feet and palms of the hands is based on the same holographic principle. For example, the holographic theory also fits well when tested by the scientific theory of DNA: every cell in the body contains information about the whole body. However, these theories are still not easy for ordinary people to understand, it is especially difficult to interpret the question raised by this specific case: why did Paida of leg reduce the thyroid lump on the neck?

Therefore, I must interpret the discussion a little in terms of the meridian theory. In the previous case discussion, we have talked many times about the location of the thyroid gland, which is where the six meridians (three Yang and three Yin meridians) of the hands pass through. How do blockages in these meridians cause their various symptoms? Blockages in the central, lung, large intestine and small intestine meridians are the most common. Is there a direct link between the six meridians and thyroid lesions? If you look at the meridians, you will find out that they are directly related. Among them, the stomach, spleen, kidney and liver meridians get through the throat directly, while the gall gallbladder and gallbladder meridians get through the neck directly. In other words, all six foot meridians get through the thyroid area. The author patted his legs for four or five hours. No matter which part of his legs he patted, he never left these six meridians, they reached the thyroid gland from different angles. It is normal to have this healing effects.

This case also bears witness to the reasons why I repeatedly advocate PL the whole body. Given the complexity of the knowledge of meridians and acupuncture points, it is difficult for the average person to grasp. You are certainly right to pat your extremities properly. If you do not have time, pat the joints of the limbs, i.e. the universal parts. There is another method, i.e. often doing head and face of Paida. Some people complain that meridians are too difficult to learn. It is one of the reasons why Chinese medicine is so difficult to learn, you cannot learn deeper. Nowadays, it is simplified with limbs and universal parts, people still can not go deeper into practice for the reason: it is too simple! In fact, the spirit is so complex!

## 2-9 The size of thyroid nodule had nearly gone after the fist Paida

I did not remember when thyroid nodule was found in my physical examination, it was just a few millimeters at first. I did not pay much attention to it. Because it is a common problem in modern times. It was only in January this year that I became aware of the nodule when it suddenly got bigger and was already quire large by the visual inspection. After I had my second child in January this year, the nodule suddenly grew in the lager size within a month, everyone asked me to have an operation.

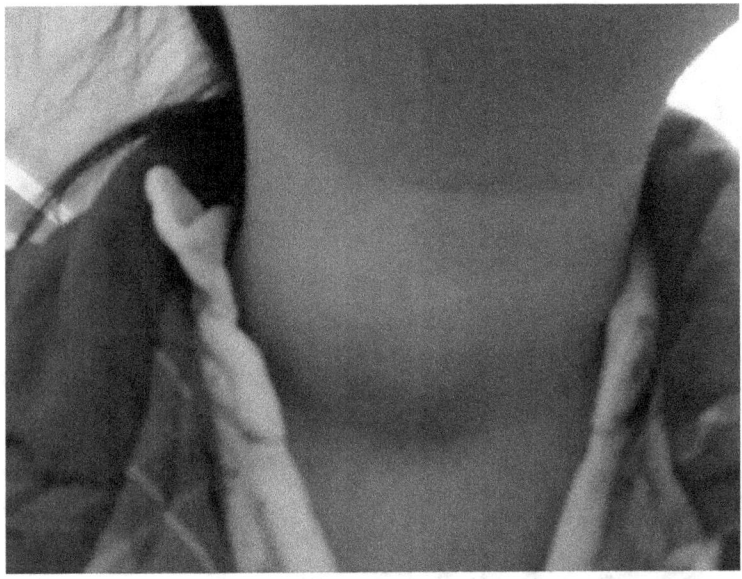

At that time, I had learned how the body heals itself and I was breastfeeding (my thyroid function was normal in the blood test at the maternity check-up), I did not go to hospital. It was my regular daily diet below: I woke up in the morning with a cup of ginger and date tea. We bought a wellness pot and brewed on a regular basis every other night, so that I could drink it ready in the morning. After the ginger and date tea comes a glass of nutritious fruit and vegetable juice, followed by breakfast as usual, I had mainly vegetarian. I must be honest. Because I had to work and take care of my kids, I really did not have much time. Therefore, it was a half-hearted effort, mainly around the thoracic spine and shoulders for about 20-30 minutes in the morning in my spare time. However, my experience is that the thyroid gland and the thymus gland are connected. I once tried Paida on the thyroid gland, there would be a feeling in the chest. I figured out that the stomach meridian passed through the thyroid gland and the chest. If it hurts to pat the chest, you can pat the thoracic spine, which also unblocked the chest and thyroid.

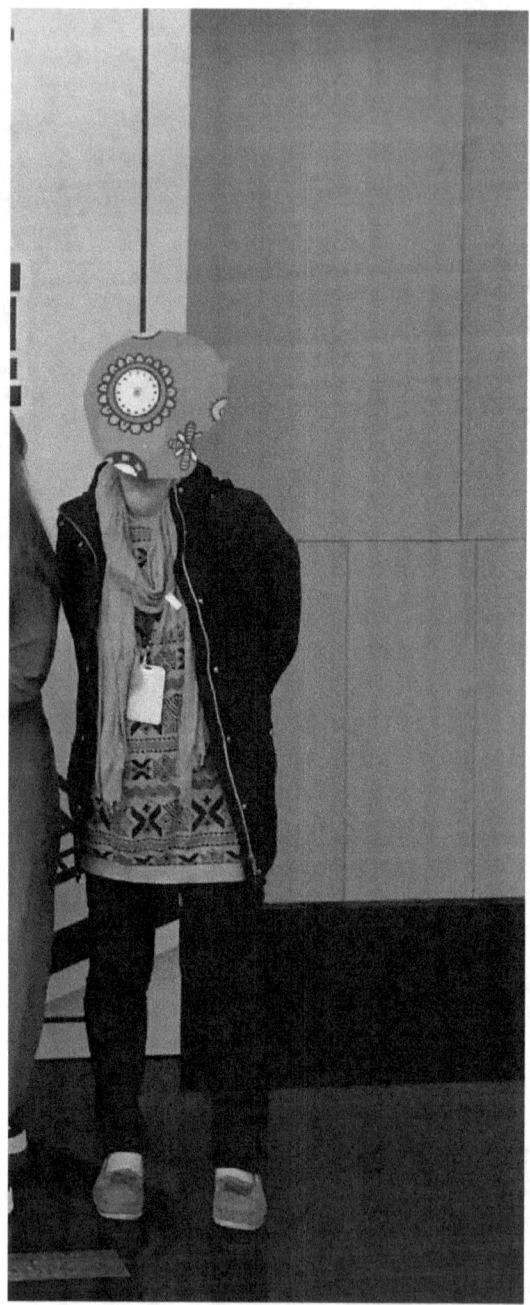

Finally, I would like to say that there should be no confrontation. I also used to fantasize about patting on the thyroid gland and its surroundings well. Maybe the nodules would disappear the next day. However, I was disappointed every time. I accepted it slowly that the oversized nodule may be accompanied with me forever, which could constantly remind me that do not get angry or lose my temper and take care of my body, then it would suddenly disappear one day.

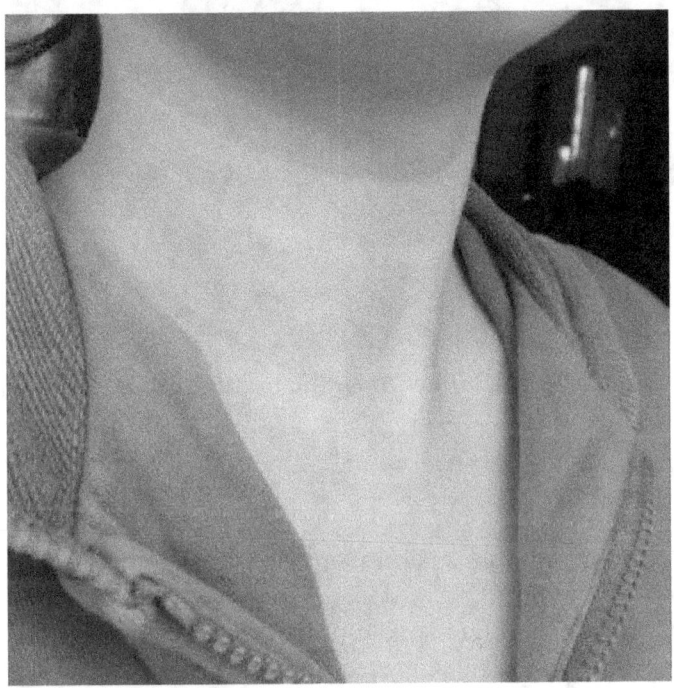

November, 2017

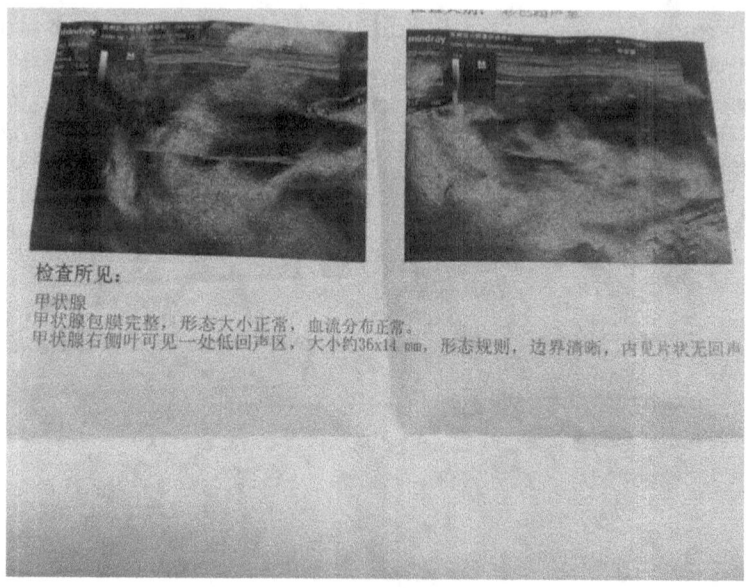

检查所见：
甲状腺
甲状腺包膜完整，形态大小正常，血流分布正常。
甲状腺右侧叶可见一处低回声区，大小约36x14 mm，形态规则，边界清晰，内见片状无回声

It was fully normal function in the body check on November 30, 2017

-- Participant from the 15th Online Camp: RBK, December 7, 2017

The thyroid nodule was present many years ago, which indicated a blockage of the associated meridians. Why did they suddenly get bigger in January? It turned out that she gave birth to her second baby by cesarean section in January. After reading the analysis of the six foot meridians in the previous case, it is easier to explore the etiology and clinical effects. The cesarean section is performed in the abdomen, which is connected to the uterus, and the meridians disrupted by the operation are the stomach, spleen, kidney and liver meridians, all four of which lead directly to the throat, which is where the thyroid gland is located. She also checked the stomach meridian route herself. Certainly, it passes through the thyroid and the chest. The chest refers to the breast, as the stomach meridian passes through the middle of the breast via the nipple. The thoracic vertebrae refers to the sternum and ribs.

The areas where she pats are mainly the sternum and ribs, which basically covers the four meridians of the stomach, spleen, liver and kidney. Another area with frequent Lajin is the shoulder, where the six meridians (three Yang and three Yin meridians) of the hands happen to be concentrated, their blockage is also the cause of thyroid disease. In particular, the heart, pericardium, lung and large intestine meridians are connected to the front and outside, which is more convenient for self-taking. In addition to the self Paida, she uses her own mindfulness: "Do not be confrontational. I accepted it slowly that the oversized nodule may be accompanied with me forever, which could constantly remind me that do not get angry or lose my temper and take care of my body, then it would suddenly disappear one day."

The mindfulness works. Because you are not making an enemy of the disease, the poor meridians caused by the fearful mind are then gradually changed by the smooth flow of meridians formed by the friendly mind. Tension and stress can lead to chronic tightening of the heart, pericardium and lung meridians, creating depression and heart disease. The combination of mindfulness and PL are helpful in opening up the meridians, so that the causes of nodule formation can gradually dissolve and the nodules naturally disappear.

The following cases are clinical experiments with more complex illnesses, and thyroid disease is only one of the complex illnesses. They have taken some wrong detours because of the complexity of disease, especially the complexity of the mood and the wrong knowledge. One of the biggest misconceptions in understanding the etiology of the disease is the lack of knowledge of the dominant role played by heart disease and cardiac disease in all diseases. The most distinctive features of two diseases are the severe blockage of the heart and pericardial meridians. The symptoms are often other more obvious or easily detectable symptoms. HC are the more obvious diagnostic marker, which can refer to as an "Energy marker", in contrast to the biomarkers used in Western medicine. It can be cross-referenced with biomarkers used in Western medicine.

Once you get used to HC and the meridians behind the various lesions to diagnose and heal yourself, healing gradually changes from a dangerous game to a joyful one. Forgetting the name of the disease and paying attention to the meridians gradually becomes a habit and an instinct.

## 2-10 Why can thyroid, pharyngitis and hepatitis B be self-healed? However, why are dizziness, insomnia and stomach problems persisting?

I attended Sensei Liu Ying's five-day workshop in Guangzhou in 2017. After the training, I followed the camp and have been patting my whole body at home on my own and have gained a lot in the past three years.

My thyroid nodules disappeared, my chronic pharyngitis cleared up, my small triple-positive hepatitis B was normalized. I also had hypertension in the past. After one year of Paida, my hypertension became low, and I left it alone. At that time, it was not like now, where the teacher can keep an eye on you and correct things at any time. When you pat yourself at home, you may just exert too much force and always be in a state of leaking.

I recently attended the two-class session. After two months of study, I still have a lot of conditions because I am old. First,, I still have stomach problems now, which was a serious problem in the past; secondly, it is still dizziness; thirdly, I can not sleep well at night, my hands and feet are cold sometimes. These are the three biggest problems bothering me now.

A few days ago when I first attended the class and asked the teacher why was I dizzy and he said that my dizziness must be solved, I spent more than two hours for Paida on my head vigorously according to the teacher's Paida method. The next day, I did Paida on my head vigorously for another two hours, and the whole body was immediately too weak to bear. My whole body became cold, I was sweating coldly and uncontrollably, and I was shivering all over. I cannot stand still.

I was ready to quit the class, I did not want to take the class anymore. However, I thought that they were HC, I could only take a break and then pat again slowly. I went along with the thought on that last day and hastily signed up for the carpet class.

I asked my teacher again, he said that it shall be patted slowly, when your body is weak, and regulate more time according to your situation. I followed the teacher's suggestion, and I basically patted for four to five hours a day, with the method of light PL, I also know by reading the book that light PL is used for tonic, heavy PL is used for drainage, my lesson was heavy PL in the past, drainage was too hard, especially when the body was weaker. The heavy PL is not suitable for the weak condition.

Under the light PL, I now feel that my burst of dizziness was getting better with each PL. Dizziness kept repeating, two or three times a day. I thought that they were also HC, which was slowly reducing the dizziness one at a time. It was impossible to release my dizziness all at once, it was working slowly.

I was desperately patting on the stomach meridian the day before yesterday because my stomach, increasingly unable to eat too much, could only eat less. When I ate less, I was particularly chilly, my body seemed to need nutrients. If I ate more, I could not enjoy it. Thus, I was determined to pat the stomach meridian. Since my feet were always cold, I chose this bone on the stomach meridian below my knees and on the Tsusanli for Paida, I did Paida as hard as I could.

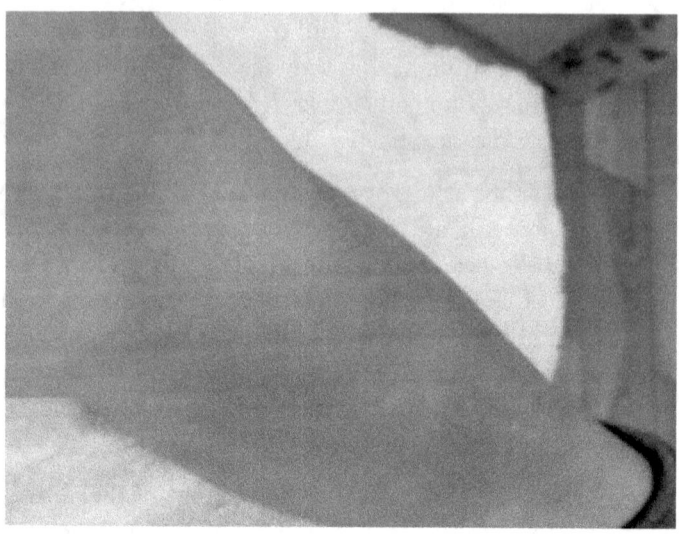

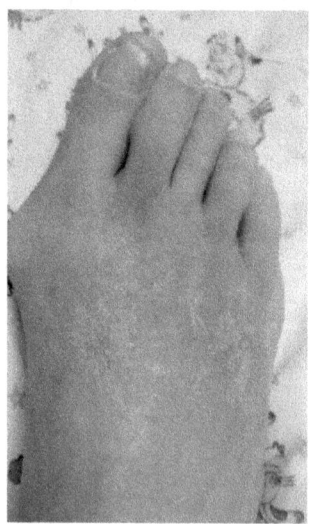

The light PL time was lengthened. During the light PL, it was painful that I could barely hold on. However, I gritted my teeth and kept going. Two days before, Paida on this bone in my left leg was conducted along the stomach meridian for four to five hours. At the morning, I also saw bruises come out, it came out last night, it was so painful in the middle of the night yesterday. I did moxibustion again at the location where the bruises came out for half an hour, so that I would slowly fell asleep. The bruises came out when I got up in the morning.

I could draw the conclusion of my experiences: the older, weaker fellows must gently pat, the bruises can come out for the long time of slow patting process, it shall take more time for the bruises to come out, do not pat with great force. Because the bruises can come out by patting bones, while skin scraping is still difficult for the bruises coming out, I believed that the bruises were coming out from bones.

Coach Liu just sent a photo when I was patting in Guangzhou, I took a big bag on my forehead, I saw that photo, Coach Liu Ying kept the information of each of us, it was really moved, the teacher ran so many classes, there were so many people, all kept the information, it encouraged me greatly, the teacher was hard, she still remembers all students. Thank you, our teachers. I will modify it myself later and have better patting on the various positions. I will come back to participate in the teacher's training class in the future.

That's all my feeling, I did not expel so many bruises as the younger sisters. However, I have gained a lot. Thank you, all teachers, especially Coach Chen and Coach Tan, who took care of us all the time.

--Yi Jing Zhi Yuan, August 5, 2020

The author patted continuously after participating in the workshop in the early days, who had healed thyroid nodules, chronic pharyngitis, and hepatitis B herself. It is more incredible that her hypertension became hypotension more than a year of PL after her early workshop. Many cases with hypertension were reduced into low blood pressure by PL. They are caused by continuing to take anti-hypertensive medication after the blood pressure was normalized. The medication was stopped at the normalized blood pressure. If the author did not take the anti-hypertensive medication and develop into hypotension, it can only mean the obvious fact that she did not recover from her heart disease. Otherwise, she did not know that her specific heart condition at all.

Her self-healed thyroid disease and pharyngitis were the result of blockages in the heart, pericardium, and lung meridians. Her throat was connected to the lung and heart meridians, which showed that her heart meridian had always been blocked. Her previous hypertension further indicated that she has heart disease. Let us look at her three worst illnesses: stomach problems, dizziness, and insomnia, all of them are also direct symptoms of a blockage in the heart meridian. Stomach problems are directly related to the heart. Because the heart is fire nature and the stomach is earth nature. Among the five elements, fire nature can produce earth nature, so that a bad heart and stomach must be sick. When people have a bad mood, be angry or depressed, it is normal to have stomach pains and lack of appetite. When the heart and pericardium meridians are blocked, the fire nature of heart is difficult to produce earth nature in the spleen and stomach, which affects digestion. From the above analysis, a simple truth shall be illustrated that: her illnesses, whether she has healed herself or not were related to heart disease.

She had chills and cold sweats after Paida of her head vigorously for two hours for two days, which is another HC of heart disease. When she does not eat or eats less, stomach chills could occur, which is also caused by a lack of heart fire, so that her stomach does not have enough stomach Qi to digest food. Originally, her chills and cold sweats were HC, which is good for her! However, fear arose in her mind that she had overshot and was leaking too hard. In fact, it is exactly the process of diagnosis and healing. The easiest way to deal with it is patting the elbow fossa and Neiguan acupoint, to open the heart and pericardium meridians up. It is a rare good sign that patting the head can produce HC of heart attack. Otherwise, she would not have known the severity of heart attack.

Another treatment increases the internal and external heat sources. The internal heat should drink ginger and date tea, while the external heat should heat to the chest and head with red bean bags and other methods. A combination of the two methods is better. It is more efficiently when the cold is drained. If you still do not understand, please ask yourself: you can expel a lot of cold energy and cold sweat from your whole body by patting your head, which means that the coldness in your heart and stomach has been here for a long time. However, you do not even know it. Would not it be great to expel the poison of cold that has been hidden for a long time now? What are HC? It is to turn out the known and unknown foci of disease in the body and expel them out of the body. A large amount of cold and dampness has been living in the heart, spleen, stomach and even the whole body for a long time, it will cause blockages in the heart, pericardium, stomach, and spleen meridians, which is the root cause of her stomach problems, dizziness, insomnia and low blood pressure. It was further analyzed that dizziness is a typical symptom of low blood pressure, which is caused by blockages in the heart and pericardium meridians in turn.

Therefore, she is not necessary to pat her head. The elbow socket, the whole inner and outer arm shall be recommended for dizziness first. Since HC of heart attack was triggered by patting the head first, it was also good, which shall just deal with it as above. Paida of the general area and limbs are always emphasized first for the stability of Paida opening, but also as a diagnosis to figure out the working meridians, it is also safer. She said that her feet were always cold, which also proven that there is a lot of coldness in her body. It is just HC for expelling cold and perspiration to release the symptom. Since it is known to be predominantly cold, in addition to the above-mentioned patting on the elbow and supplementing internal and external heat sources, hot water to soak the feet can be also suggested. The feet and legs were patted after soaking them to produce bruises more quickly. The stomach meridian and spleen meridian is located on the legs and feet, so that stomach problems can be dissolved quickly after Paida through the meridians. Chinese medicine talks about two major causes of insomnia: (1) Lack of intercourse between the heart and kidneys; (2) Disharmony between the spleen and stomach. These conditions are related to the inability of the heart meridian.

It seemed that forgetting the name of the disease is easier said than done. In this case, it did not necessarily start Paida of head for the dizziness and Paida of the stomach meridian for the stomach disorders first. Paida of the heart and pericardium meridians are combined with the internal and external heat sources and feet soaking, which shall be first recommended. Besides, she did not mention Lajin. Lajin is also a good overall method for clearing the meridians as well as a tonic method for draining cold out of the body. She was distracted, fearful and suspicious during HC, which drained the cold inside the body. It was actually HC for anxiety, rather than a discharge. If the poison of cold is discharged, it means that it exactly should be drained, which is the advantage of HC. However, once HC happens to the individual, people could be frightened, so that they could forget its advantages and benefits, even they could forget HC!

It is concluded that her previous self-healing thyroid disease, pharyngitis and hepatitis was mainly caused by the fact that the heart and lung meridians had been opened up partly, rather than opened up completely. Especially, because the cold had not been expelled and the heart and stomach were blocked in the cold. Therefore, the symptoms of stomach problems, dizziness, insomnia and low blood pressure could occur. As for this case, HC not only brought out the coldness of heart disease and stomach trouble, but also flushed out her heart disease, which indicated that she had not yet truly understood the inner meaning of HC in her cognition. Fear was not caused by the external phenomena. However, your interpretation of the phenomena, and your interpretation depends on your knowledge, i.e. your thoughts. Therefore, it shall be corrected the knowledge at its source. Because thoughts and ideas exist in the mind, which is under the command of the mind. Thus, the destiny of the body is determined by the mind.

## 2-11 Menopausal hot flashes, heartburn, insomnia, thyroid tumor and heart disease

I had a unhealthy body from my childhood, and I was often ill. Later, I got lymphatic tuberculosis at university. During the treatment, I was infected by a blind puncture by the university physician, which almost killed me. During the treatment, I took a lot of western medicine, my poor health even became worse.

Headaches, dizziness and colds became my norm during working, and I took a lot of medicine. However, my health did not improve. In the year of my doctoral studies, a thyroid tumor was detected during a physical examination, and I started to take Chinese medicine again. I knew that I had the serious heart problem. Because I would have cardiac convulsion during naps and at night, like chills. However, the equipment could not detect them yet. Once they were detected, I believe that the disease will not be able to heal.

Since then, I have been practicing food therapy, learning moxibustion, massage, and exploring various health care methods. In 2014, I went to the US for a year and returned with Hashimoto's thyroiditis and enlarged thyroid nodules. Meanwhile, there were several cases of highly educated people who died young for fatal illnesses and heart attacks at the school, including my colleagues.

I began to wonder if there was any point in continuing to pursue a career at the expense of my body. Should I quit? Or should I stay on? The people can be impossible to stop for the pressure of research and teaching, and the pursuit is endless! In 2017, I was finally approved to retire from active service, which was the end of my career!

Since then, I have been free from the burden of scientific research everyday, then I devoted myself to studying methods of nourishing and regulating the body: learning the classics of Chinese medicine, moxibustion, acupuncture, massage, and scraping. The methods used were effective at first, a noticeable improvement in my body could be seen. After half a month, they were no longer effective. The insomnia was getting worse and I could hardly sleep at night. During this period, I practiced Hubei Kaoshan Kongfu, it was similar to PL, and my heart problems were improved. However, my insomnia still had not improved.

In the summer of 2018, someone in a group shared an article on PL, so that I followed PL's public website. It was also in this summer that I patted myself on my arms and legs. At that time, there was full of big bruises after Paida. As I did not know the specific reason for bruises, I patted them and left them alone, and it took more than 10 days for them to recede. After two or three times, I never did it again. I did keep patting my head for a long time. Paida was only used for health purposes without enough strengths. Therefore, after Paida on the head, my headache and insomnia improved. While the headache recurred frequently without the long effectiveness.

I bought the stretching bench in the autumn of 2018 and put it away after just a few stretches without any encouragement when I first started to stretch under the intolerable pain. Thus, Lajin was stopped until October 2020!

In April and May 2020, I started to experience menopausal hot flushes. Almost every few minutes, my body suddenly become hot and sweaty. At first, it was worked for the medication. Later, the medication did not work either. I was already extremely sick in October.

One night, before I went to bed, my stomach started to burn again and I remembered to pat Tsusanli from PL class, so I patted on the left foot with a tool and the bruises kept coming out. After a few minutes, my stomach had eased. I could sleep well without taking any medication that night. Since then, I have stopped taking my stomach medication!

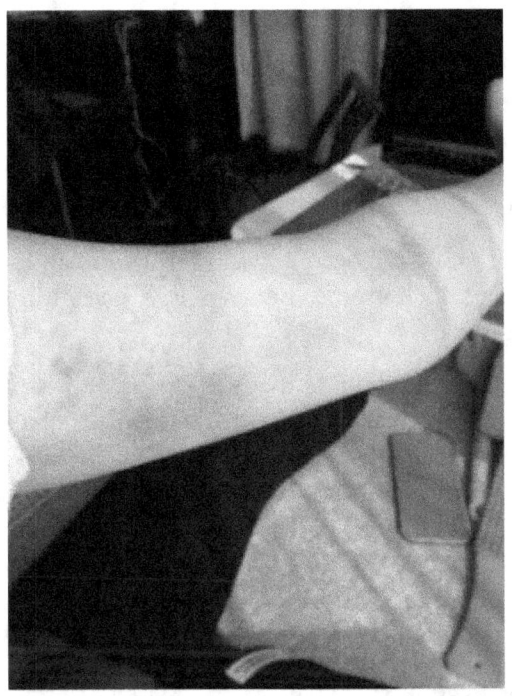

    I am grateful to Coach Liu Ying and Coach Xiao Tian for their enthusiastic guidance! Since then, I have been practicing PL seriously, stretching every morning and evening in the lying position. After a week of straining and patting the painful areas, I suddenly noticed: the menopausal hot flushes disappeared unnoticed. I continued to pat, and the large bruises all over my arms and legs. Slowly, after lying down at 10:00 pm, I was able to fall asleep quickly. Although I kept waking up, it was better than the previous torment of restlessness and sleepless nights.

    During the process of PL, the bloating that used to plague me all year round (in the afternoon I would bulge from my lower left abdomen and a surge of Qi would go up to my chest compartment without releasing, which was quite unpleasant and lasted until 7:00 pm or 8:00 pm) was also gradually relieved. Over the past few years, I have had scary varicose veins under my tongue, which indicated the result of severe blockage of meridians in my body.

After few months of PL, especially the recent 3-hour continuous bombardment and online carpet bombardment, I had noticed that the reef-like clusters of veins under my tongue had been shrunk significantly, which meant that when the meridians were gradually being cleared, the pressure on the veins to return was slowly decreasing.

In the last 4 months, I have been adhering to PL, I can feel that the thyroid tumor, which used to be very large, has shrunk significantly by touching.

In the past, I had regulated my body by the various methods, the bad effectiveness shown was not the wrong methods taken. Because my body was so badly blocked that the medicine was not effective enough to get through. Moxibustion for the five centers were even more of a result of the severe stasis blockage. There is no quicker and more effective way to solve the stasis in the body other than PL! Although there are still some unresolved issues, I believe that the path of PL will only get better and better!

I am grateful for meeting PL. Thanks, Mr. Xiao, Coach Liu Ying, and the loving family of PL!!

--Hui Huige, 2021.3.6

It is another symphonic tragedy with heart disease as the main theme. It is even sadder that heart disease is present throughout her medical history and her various medical conditions, to the extent that heart spasms become the norm, while medical examinations always say that her heart is normal. "I know that there is serious problems in my heart. Because there were heart spasms with chills during naps and at night, which had just not detectable by the instruments yet. Once it is detected, I believe that the disease will not be able to heal."

Her self-diagnosis was indeed accurate. Midday, at 11:00-13:00 pm, is the time of heart meridian. Therefore, heart spasms during siesta is evidence of a serious heart condition. Among the list of conditions directly related to heart disease include headache, dizziness, insomnia, thyroid tumor, thyroiditis and lymphatic tuberculosis. They are directly related because they are the direct result of blockages in the heart and pericardial meridian. Symptoms related to the heart indirectly are menopausal hot flushes, heartburn, bloating and colds. How do you get these illnesses? According to Western medicine, it is so-called a malfunctioning immune system. Why is it malfunctioning?

It can be concluded that the history of treatment is the result of taking medication. First, she had lymphatic tuberculosis, which nearly killed her with a puncture. "I took a lot of Western medicine during treatment, which aggravated my poor health. After work, headaches, dizziness, and colds became the norm, and I ate handfuls of medicines. However, my body did not get better. In the year of my doctoral studies, a thyroid tumor was detected during a physical examination, and I started to take Chinese medicine again. Insomnia, bloating and abnormal heart spasms started to become the new norm slowly..." As a result, she was forced to stop working and focus on her medical treatment.

She had originally learned to PL in 2018. While she stopped after two or three times, and the stretching bench was bought and used a few times for fear of pain, which was not used again. Two years were wasted, that is, she suffered two years of sickness and pain. The bruises and pain suffered were HC, which was a good sign for diagnosis and healing. Why did she stop PL? It is typical HC of heart disease, where doubts and fears conquer her. Doubt and fear originated from her knowledge. As a scholar, she has studied *Theory of Paida* and conducted serious clinical trials before making a judgement. However, she easily interpreted a HC with her past knowledge, which showed that she did not really understand the basic principles of Paida and did not conduct in-depth clinical trials, and she only used it superficially.

Later, when her menopausal hot flushes appeared, she had used all natural treatments such as acupuncture, scraping and moxibustion, all of them were not valid. The heartburn and insomnia attacked again; lasting half a year before she finally patted on the Tsusanli of the stomach meridian at night. In just a few minutes the stomach symptoms disappeared, "I did not take any medication this night and I could fall into sleep by the method actually. After that, my stomach medication was completely stopped!" It was a forced clinical experiment of Paida, a sickness forcing a spiritual transformation. In fact, it is the real meaning of being sick.

After that she began "to practice PL seriously, every morning and evening in the lying position. While stretching, she patted on the painful areas." It was at this point that her interpretation of pain had changed, a change of heart. So just a week after PL, the hot flushes disappeared. "I continued to Paida along with big bruises all over the arms and legs slowly. After lying down at 10:00 pm, I was actually able to fall asleep quickly." With the remarkable clinical results, whether the disease was healed by PL or her heart? Clearly, the real healer is her mind. PL was just a method or a tool, it was so simple. She had to change her mind and all healing effects appeared.

In fact, there were so many bruises all over her body, which meant that all the meridians were blocked, which were worst and critical blockages of the heart, pericardium, and lung meridians. Since all the meridians were blocked, what better way to open them than PL? She had been doing clinical trials with the rest of the methods and medicines by herself for over ten years and she knew the results clearly. Why could the abdominal distension symptoms be improved, the sublingual venous plexus be improved, and the thyroid tumor be significantly reduced by simple PL? It was clearly the result of the meridians throughout the body being unblocked. A complex combination of illnesses for decades was finally simply concluded as meridian blockage, which can be solved by PL. Among these meridians, the unblocking heart and pericardium meridians can play a decisive role. Once the heart functions are normal, insomnia, hot flushes, thyroid, and other unexplained symptoms would be improved naturally. How do we know that her heart and pericardial meridians had been opened up? Were the improvement on these symptoms and bruises all over her arms and legs also the excellent verification of HC?

She had already started PL on her whole body. She was still patting herself. It could be better if she joins the mutual Paida actions and attends an offline workshop, her whole physical and mental state will go to the next level. If she pats on her hands, feet and head with more bruises, the improvement of her illness will also be accelerated, which means that the meridians associated with the heart and brain will be opened up more thoroughly. However, the time and intensity of Paida depends on the decision of her mind. Her mind obviously had to change.

## 2-12 Total improvement of dry syndrome, thyroid nodules, heart disease and depression

As the seven-day PL experience was almost over, my body had been relaxed, my mood was happy and my heart felt better. Although I still had vague pains in the areas after Paida, I felt that it had been well worth.

My health was improved as below:

Firstly: my mouth is not dry anymore. I can talk and read aloud for an hour without drinking any water. Previously, I went to hospital for a check-up because I had little saliva in my mouth and was diagnosed with dryness syndrome in the past. The doctor said that I had an immune system disorder with an unknown cause and no specific medicine. When I asked them what the consequences would be, the doctor said that if the disease continued to develop, the eyes, the mouth and the nose would be dry, the body would not sweat, and the disorders of organs would occur due to the lack of body fluids, and the body would become a veritable "mummy" eventually. In July 2015, I attended PL camp, and I was able to see immediate results in 3-5 minutes of Paida. It was amazing! After several times of PL on the hands, face and mouth, you could obtain the instant results and save money. What a wonderful experience! The effect was even more pronounced with a longer PL.

Secondly, I was found to have multiple thyroid nodules on both sides in 2014, with the largest one as 5.7mm. At the end of the workshop in July 2015, the nodules were only found on one side with only 3.4mm. I believe that the nodules will disappear after PL.

Thirdly, I had a heart condition, it was not detected in the physical examination. When it is cold, my lips are usually purple. On the first day of Paida, a blood blister came out. The instructor said that the heart disease was tuned out and healed by PL, I was so happy.

Fourthly, after Paida of my breasts, the bruises came out miserably with the intense pain. After Paida, it was comfortable. It seemed that years of suppressed aggression were swept away, it was so painful.

In 2016, I would hope that my white hair would turn into black. I would be happy to stop dying my hair; I shared PL with more people; I could have the opportunity to volunteer at the camp; and I will set up a PL supporting group.

I am grateful to our coaches and friends. We were centered by PL. If we have the right concept of health and adhere to PL forever. We believe that health and happiness will always be with us.

-- Ms. Jiang 26-02-2016

This case is a summary of the two workshops. The four conditions listed by the author for improvement are all directly related to heart meridian disorders, although the names of the conditions are different. Dry syndrome and thyroid disease may develop as endocrine disorders. However, they are also essentially complications of heart disease. One might even say that the heart, the largest endocrine organ, is also the largest immune organ.

Let's talk about dry syndrome first. Doctors said that it was an immune system disease, the cause is unknown, and it is not healed. Why did PL of the hands, face and mouth work immediately to produce saliva? It is the result of opening up the meridians and HC. The heart, pericardium and lung meridians locate on the palms and inner arms, which passes through the heart and lungs in the chest; the large intestine, small intestine and San Jiao meridians locate on the back of the hands and outer arms, which pass through head and face, as well as the large and small intestines in the abdomen. The large intestine meridian penetrates more directly into the lips and gums of the mouth, and the small intestine meridian passes through the side of the face. Face, lips, gums and mouth are also densely distributed by the stomach and large intestine meridians. Paida on these areas opens up and stimulates the heart meridian, stomach meridian, large intestine meridian and small intestine meridian. The so-called endocrine disorders indicate that these meridians are not working. When they are opened up, they return to normal. Its central meridian is the most crucial, as it connects the throat and brain. Therefore, the whole body's nervous system is connected to the brain, which is one of the reasons that the brain is considered the largest immune organ.

As for thyroid disease. In the previous case discussions, I have repeatedly pointed out that the thyroid location converges the six meridians from the hand, namely the heart, pericardium, lung, large intestine, small intestine, and San Jiao meridians. Besides, the thyroid gland is also connected to the six foot meridians of the stomach, spleen, kidney and liver. It can be found that these meridians are almost identical to those that cause dryness syndrome. It is still the heart, large intestine and stomach meridians that play a key role. All kinds of immune system and endocrine disorders are just blockages in these meridians, which can be cleared up. If you do not understand the meridian system, just pat your limbs and head and face to basically resolve your illnesses. Of course, it is better to pat the whole body thoroughly and combine with Lajin.

Thirdly, let us talk about heart disease. It is the most difficult disease to diagnose in Western medicine and it is easiest to diagnose with Paida. You can find out by Paida on the heart of the elbow socket and the pericardial meridian. Heart disease sounds scary, while it is not actually. Because it is just a blockage of the heart and pericardium meridians, which can be opened. In fact, patients with heart disease are caused by the blocked heart and pericardial meridians, with a different extent for the different patients. Heart disease can be easy and effective to treat by Paida, so that it is not scary. It is scary that you are oblivious to its symptoms and complications. For example, dry syndrome, thyroid disease, hypertension or headaches, dizziness, insomnia, weakness and other symptoms stem from blockages in the heart meridian. For example, the blood blisters after Paida on the heart meridian are an excellent HC, which dissolves the heart disease and improves all the complications.

Fourthly, let us talk about breast diseases. We can see many cases in the Clinical Discussion of Breast Diseases from the *Clinical Report on Gynecological Diseases PL*. Although the case did not point out the specific condition of breast, it is the fact that the bruises of breast are so disastrous, which indicates that the meridians are severely blocked. The meridians connected to the breast are basically the same as those that cause many chronic diseases, including thyroid disease and dryness syndrome, namely the heart, pericardium, lung, stomach, liver, spleen, and kidney. Therefore, it seemed that Paida of breast is not only self-healing for breast disease, but it is also associated with improvements in many conditions. Why did she feel so comfortable after Paida of her breast, as if all the grievances that she had suppressed for years had been swept away? Because Paida of breast opens the heart and pericardium meridians. The symptoms of depression are manifested in the meridians as blockages in the heart and pericardium meridians, so it is natural to feel better after opening them up.

Based on the discussion of this case, we could have further insight into why we should forget the name of the illness and focus on the clearing of the meridians. Because the name of disease is only an appearance, and different names are just different manifestations of the same meridian blockage. The clinical and theoretical aspects of PL are constantly verified to the fact that meridian failure is the essential cause of all diseases. Therefore, we shall learn to figure out the essence through phenomena by PL.

## 2-13 A dozen diseases can be healed by PL

Hello, everyone! My name is Liu Yanxia. It is a fact that the sequelae of blood clots of 73-year-old grandmother was healed by her granddaughter with Paida for three months. I saw the happiness of the old woman after she was healed!

The granddaughter did not go to work for three months to fulfill her filial piety for her mother, which is filial piety. Thus, her grandmother was able to stop suffering from her illness! Paida process was only option at the time! However, since I spread the method, her family took it seriously, so that she obtained unexpected results! It has relieved several generations of troubles!

The 73-year-old women stumbledes on her feet. It was so difficult; she had survived now! She got better with the careful Paida by her family. Filial piety and faith was really moving! At present, the elderly is living in the nursing house, her daughter hires a care worker to continue Paida for her. My friend - Liang Liping (her daughter) is unable to help her. Because her mother-in-law is ill and serve her for better living quality. We should learn from the virtues of their families. It is no doubt about PL. Just trust it!

Today, I would share my own story. Thanks to PL, I have changed from a painful experience to the happy one, which is a long story!

Some years ago, I used my own farm vehicle for selling fertilizer, rice and so on. Because of the tiredness of the work, I once fell and hurt my left side and the load on my right side was so heavy that it caused a herniated disc in my lower back. My back hurt, and my right shoulder blade felt like it had been stabbed with an awl, so I knocked on it by a rolling pin. The pain was so bad that I had to go to hospital for injections and medication. Later, an orthopedic surgeon said, "If you break it, I can put it back together to ensure that you will never break it again or have any more problems. However, it cannot be returned back again if the bone is stretched out. It is not easy, the membrane can not wrap around the bone, it is a permanent scar, you are disabled for entire life." It is so desperate; it becomes lumbar disc herniation. I asked the doctor what should I do? He said that the only way shall be nursing.

When I got home, I could not move, my herniated disc got worse, and I hit my back with a rolling pin when the pain became serious. When I returned home, I continued to conduct the fluid infusion and take Chinese medicine. I was paralyzed before long. At that time, the herbal medication increased my white blood cells and my periods turned white and all of them flowing out was white.

Misfortunes never come singly. Illness has come in groups to torture me. After that, I had thyroid nodules, lymph nodules, muscle atrophy...

Later, the second uncle of my eldest sister (a doctor) conducted a CT test for me, a full body check-up and found lumbar spinal stenosis, he said, "Auntie, do not take medicine. If you take medicine again, you will kill yourself. The herniated disc can not be treated, you can only massage it. If it gets any worse, you should have surgery. Massage is suggested." Since my second sister also told me that overtaking Diclofenac would lead to osteoporosis, I did not dare to take the medicine again. When I returned, I had to continue to take Chinese herbs plus vitamin B1 and B6. From 34 years old to 50 years old, I was tormented for more than 10 years! Anyway, I was worse as a living death at that time! I often had the suicidal thought! I was sick of it!

I hit the elbow fossa first and the heart stopped hurting, I had all eight general areas did Lajin. My heels hurt, but they did not hurt after Paida either. Later in the dojo, Ms. Fan Guangqin patted my left leg because my left leg was numb all the time; Senior Zhou Hongye patted my chest and back. I had a serious HC when I patted my breast.

My proper Paida was only the one time that I went to the dojo. Since I went to work, I just tried to see if my leg would work or not, and the result proved: Yes! All these symptoms that I had before are gone, and the muscle atrophy in my arms at that time is gone now. I can take my grandchildren to the nursery school; I can dance with my sisters. I am completely recovered in healthy condition, as a normal person. What a miracle!

**Improvements after PL:**

Three breast nodules had gone.

One of three fibroid was left and two fibroids had gone.

Two thyroid nodules had gone.

Lymph nodules had gone.

Blurred vision had restored to 1.4 or 1.5.

Fatty liver had gone, and the weight returned to normal with the weight loss.

There was something on the vitreous humour of the eye. The doctor said that we could not treat it. If it was treated, I could go blind. Moreover, my eyes might fall out if I was blinking! Is it true? While the black mass is now gone when the eye is moved.

Pyloric enlargement had gone.

Duodenal ulcers were healed.

Cervical spondylosis was healed.

High uric acid became normal!

Muscle atrophy in the right arm was restored!

Scapulohumeral periarthritis had gone!

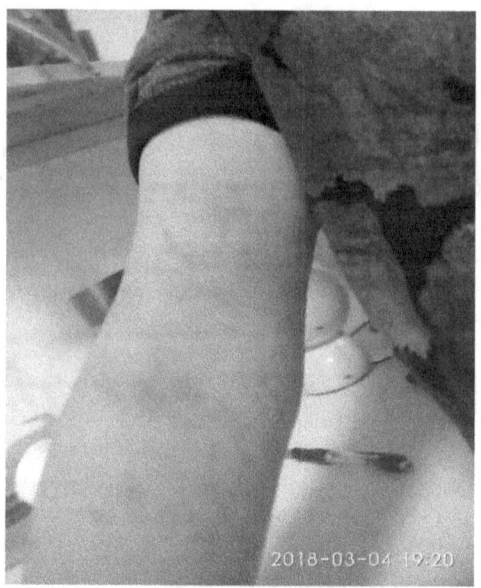

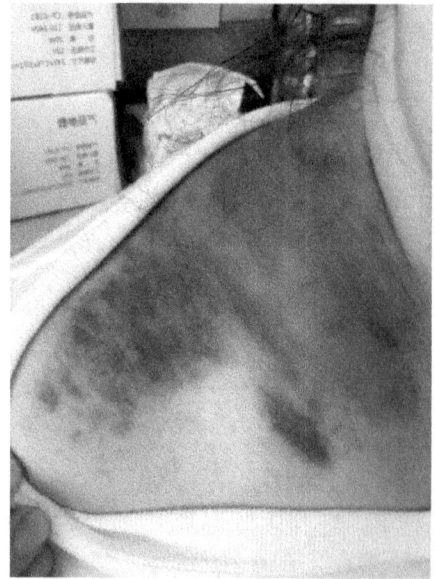

    My formal contact with PL started when Mr. Zhang Shuangwen established a group in May 2017. In the past, PL was purely a solution. When I was paralyzed, my stomach was full of air, my body was full of air and I had nowhere to vent the feeling that it would be good if there were vertebrae or needles stuck in my back to release air. Thus, I patted myself with a rolling pin and burped, I was very comfortable.

Since the medication had already caused other serious adverse reactions, I started to pat systematically after I entered the group to learn. For example, if your elbow hurts, your heel hurts, you should pat on the general area, such as your shoulder and others. More tears will be shed for touching! Traditional culture and PL are life-savers. I never want to give up after it had been grabbed!

Dear families, please believe in karma, grasp the straw. There is rebirth and ascension to higher realms by following the teacher! I can only say that the details are too convoluted, and the desire can be healed with medicine lasted for years and it was slipped out through the torment of needles and medicine! At present, I can jump and dance! I can work again! I can run up and down the stairs, and I can load 25 Kg of goods up to the fifth floor with two hands without taking a break, which is not very breathless!

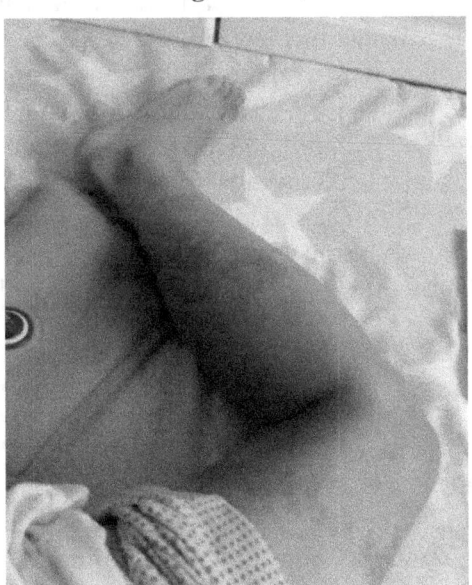

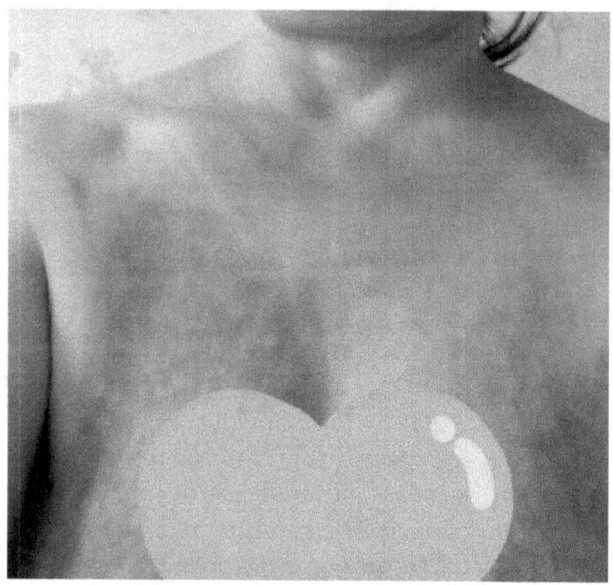

The greatest benefit was also learning about traditional culture under the guidance of Mr. Zhang Shuangwen's brother, Mr. Zhang Jingping. In the atmosphere of traditional culture, it is like a fish in water, people can be able to read and share books even over 60 years old! They are so thankful, touched, and grateful for the resurrection of the "dead". I feel like a child again. Let us follow in the footsteps of our teacher and health can be accompanied with us! Nowadays, my whole family is acting, even though they are not as hardworking as Liang Liping! Let's pat hard and heal ourselves, let's do it together! Fighting.

I have been fortunate enough to come across PL, it is a blessing to come. Thus, the family members in the group should seriously realize the importance of PL, start with me. Let the love spread on earth. A word spreads so that more people can benefit: PL is an effective self-healing method, a great way to heal yourself without spending money! What are you still hesitating about? I am grateful to Mr. Zhang Shuangwen for his aerial platform, which has benefited individuals and warmed a lot of people!

After I had patted myself down, I started to mobilize my friends and family to do it. My own second brother had a bad condition in his stomach and heart, and my second sister-in-law had asthma with a lot of old problems, white bruises came out after their PL. They are all healed by PL.

Thanks, Mr. Xiao, Mr. Zhang Shuangwen and Mr. Mo Fei! It's great to follow your loving and caring teachers and seniors to make progress together! I am grateful to the families who met in the group for PL, we had obtained the benefit from it, act as a good example to relieve more people of their worries and practice! I am grateful for the encounter! I am also grateful for the example set by the practicing power from my friend Liping! I am grateful to everything!

--Author: Liu Yanxia September 2020

The author not only healed herself, but also promoted PL. The article mentioned that "A 73-year-old grandmother was healed by her granddaughter with PL for three months" in PL Clinical Report on Stroke. The author listed 13 diseases herself, plus the self-healed synovitis of the legs, herniated discs, as well as two biggest diseases: heart disease and depression, which had healed themselves, in a total of 17 diseases. Among these serious conditions, breast nodules and thyroid nodules are no longer considered to be major illnesses. Therefore, these diseases can be dissolved naturally by PL of the whole body. As you can see from the symptoms listed, she had many foreign masses for the blocked meridians and the negative effects of medication: 3 breast nodules, 3 fibroids, 2 thyroid nodules and 1 lymph nodule. How can these masses be effectively resolved with medication? The causes of the breast nodules, thyroid nodules and lymph nodules were caused by basically the same reason: the heart, lung and pericardium meridians were all blocked, so that her worst illnesses were heart disease and depression, which neither she nor her doctor knew about.

Although depression was not diagnosed, her symptoms were obvious. She wrote, "Anyway, I was worse as a living death at that time!!! I often had the suicidal thought! I was sick of it!" For 16 years, from 34 years old to 50 years old, she was treated with medication, which was one of the reasons for the increasing number of illnesses. The dozen illnesses were obviously not onset in a single day, the negative effects can be imagined that her periods turned white after taking the medication. Who could not be depressed with many illnesses simultaneously?

Depression is caused by the blocked heart meridian. When it is blocked for a long time, heart disease can be developed. She said that she conducted Paida of the heart at the first time, she "tapped on the elbow socket first, and the pain in the heart eased." Her heart had been in a state of chronic pain, which meant that heart disease was serious. "Then I did Paida of all eight general parts." However, one of her most effective Paida was a reciprocal one, "A severe HC was shown after Paida of the breast. "The so-called severe systems generally refer to dizziness, chest tightness, palpitation, and even coma, which is HC of heart disease. The inside of breast is located at the heart meridian, the pericardium meridian, and others. The heart is under the breast. It was about the only time for Paida of her breasts.

Who would have thought that Paida of breast could trigger a serious heart attack HC? Would not this just clinically validate the relationship between heart disease and breast disease? Breast nodules and thyroid nodules are caused by the same causes; they are both associated with incompetence of the heart, pericardium, and lung meridians. Moreover, they are associated with negative emotions.

# Appendix 1: Statistical Results of the Return Visits for the workshop

We made a telephone return visit in August 2011 and December 2015 to the trainees participating in the mainland workshop, and the statistical results are as follows:

### I Respondent number

There are 938 trainees listed in the return visits excluding the factor of repetition training.

### II Successful return visit number

We made the return visits with 684 persons successfully, 73% of the number of return visits should be accepted. But we failed to reach 254 persons because: 1. it was inconvenient to use phone calls to contact overseas students attending the mainland workshop ; 2. we failed to reach them because the phone number was wrong; 3. No one answered the phone.

### III Telephone return visit results

( i ) Persistence of PL

533 people among the 684 students in the successful return visits still insist on PL after returning home, 78% of the return visit number. The other 151 do not persist in PL, accounting for 22 %. The major reasons are as follows:
1. Business and full occupation.
2. Self-awareness of no disease.
3. Laziness ;
4. fear of pain.

( ii ) Drug taking conditions of trainees insisting on PL

95% of the 533 individuals who insist on PL, that is, 507 people, no longer take or have never taken any drugs. And 5 % of them, that is, 26 people, still take drugs because:
1. Serious ill patients or the elderly, fearing that their diseases can not be controlled only by PL ;

2. The doctors charge them to take medicine as a task;
3. The index fluctuates (such as high blood pressure);
4. They worry about that the disease will repeat after drug withdrawal or after complete drug withdrawal.
5. They think that the effect of combining taking drugs with PL is better.

(ⅲ) Health conditions of students who insist on PL and no longer take drugs

298 of the 507 students who insist on not taking the medication (accounting for 59%) are in good health. 172 people (accounting for 34%) have a significant improvement in their health status. 37 (accounting for 7%) remain the health condition of taking drugs and show no deterioration from withdrawal. Students in good health basically insist on PL every day with running. The higher the frequency of PL, the more prominent the effect of health improvement.

(ⅳ) Statistics of the self-healing effect of a single disease

We made separate data statistics in December 2015 of 520 people who participated in the 7-day workshop in mainland China. Six diseases have the most prominent effect (easy to test): hypertension, heart disease, diabetes, shoulder, neck and back disease, lumbar and leg pain, and joint disease, with results shown as follows:

Statistical results at the end of the 7-day workshop

| Disease | Proportion of the number of participants | Number of people | Effective number | Effective percentage |
| --- | --- | --- | --- | --- |
| Hypertension | 12% | 62 | 60 | 97% |
| Heart disease | 24% | 123 | 118 | 96% |
| Diabetes | 6% | 31 | 28 | 90% |
| Shoulder, | 56% | 292 | 265 | 91% |

| neck and back pain | | | | |
|---|---|---|---|---|
| Pain in waist and lower extremities | 42% | 220 | 203 | 92% |
| Arthronosos | 26% | 133 | 125 | 94% |

We made separate statistics on hypertension, diabetes, as well as pain in waist and lower extremities among the 684 people with whom we made these two successful return visits with results shown as follows :

1. The number of individuals with hypertension is 82, or 12% of the total number of the respondent trainees with successful visits (684). Among them, 64 (78%) have significant effect and 18 (22%) have average effect. The 18 people with average effect only occasionally practice PL, and sometimes take medicine.
2. The number of individuals with diabetes is 32, 5% of the total number of the respondent trainees with successful visits (684). Among them, 22 (69%) have significant effect while 10 (31%) have average effect.
3. The number of individuals with pain in waist and lower extremities is 234, accounting for 34% of the total number of the respondent trainees with successful visits (684). Among them, 187 (80%) have obvious effect and 47 (20%) have average effect.

Among the 399 people with whom we made successful return visits in December 2015, we added separate statistics on three diseases, that is, heart disease, shoulder, neck and back disease, and arthronosos:

1. The number of individuals with heart disease is 93, accounting for 23% of the total number of the respondent trainees with successful visits (399). Among them, 71 (76%) have obvious effect, 20 (22%) have average effect

while 2 (2%) have deterioration. And the deterioration result came out because of the severe symptoms appeared on 2 after they returned from the workshop. We had told them that it was the HC, and suggested to continue PL, but they felt that HC meant deterioration.
2. The number of individuals with neck, shoulder and back pain is 202, accounting for 51% of the total number of the respondent trainees with successful visits (399 students). Among them, 151 (75%) have a significant effect, and 51 (25%) have an average effect.
3. The number of individuals with arthronosos is 84, accounting for 21% of the total number of the respondent trainees with successful visits (399). Among them, 58 (69%) have an obvious effect, and 26 (31%) have an average effect.

## IV Summary of the return visit statistics

1. It is effective for more than 90% of the trainees who have hypertension, heart disease, diabetes, shoulder, neck and back disease, waist, and leg pain, arthronosos and other major diseases after the trainees took part in the workshop with PL practice.
2. After the students return home, so long as they insist on PL, their health will be improved significantly. It has an apparent effect for more than 69 % of people suffering from major diseases, such as hypertension, heart disease, diabetes disease, shoulder, neck and back pain, and arthronosos.
3. Among those who insist on PL, 95% (507) no longer take or have never taken any medicine. Wherein, 93 % of them are in good health and have no deterioration.

——Promotion team of PL, in January, 2016

# Appendix 2: Statistical data analysis of PL (2018)

We have received a total of 137 pieces of feedback online from June 16 to-August 20, 2018, and the specific statistics are as follows:

## 1. Gender ratio

Female: male =115:22. The number of females who practice PL is five times as that of men, indicating that women are more concerned about health than men.

## 2. Overall efficiency of PL

The overall efficiency of improving health with PL in the 137 feedback forms is 92%, and the effect of 8% is not obvious. It is mainly related to the frequency and duration of PL.

## 3. Efficiency statistics for individual conditions

The main health problems of the 137 netizens involve more than 18 kinds of diseases such as heart disease, diabetes, cervical spondylosis and periarthritis of shoulder, among which sub-health and periarthritis of shoulder account for the largest proportion, which is estimated to be related to the fast pace of life, improper daily use of computer posture and cold and other factors.

Table of self-healing efficiency for individual diseases

| Disease | Number of people | Effective number | Effective percentage | Invalid number | Inefficiency |
|---|---|---|---|---|---|
| Heart disease | 22 | 21 | 95.5% | 1 | 4.5% |
| Diabetes | 9 | 8 | 88.9% | 1 | 11.1% |
| Cervical spondylopathy | 44 | 42 | 95.5% | 2 | 4.5% |
| Scapulohumer | 50 | 47 | 94% | 3 | 6% |

| | | | | | |
|---|---|---|---|---|---|
| al periarthritis | | | | | |
| Obesity | 16 | 16 | 100% | 0 | 0 |
| Insomnia | 39 | 35 | 90% | 4 | 10% |
| Nasitis | 23 | 20 | 87% | 3 | 13% |
| Skin sensibility | 20 | 19 | 95% | 1 | 5% |
| Androgynaecology | 25 | 24 | 96% | 1 | 4% |
| Apoplexia | 1 | 1 | 100% | 0 | 0 |
| Depression | 19 | 18 | 94.7% | 1 | 5.3% |
| Sub-health | 68 | 65 | 95.6% | 3 | 4.4% |
| Dizziness and headache | 27 | 26 | 96.3% | 1 | 3.7% |
| Blood pressure problem | 18 | 18 | 100% | 0 | 0 |
| Algomenorrhea | 15 | 14 | 93.3% | 1 | 6.7% |
| Rheumatoid arthritis | 6 | 5 | 83.3% | 1 | 16.7% |
| Pain | 24 | 23 | 95.8% | 1 | 4.2% |
| Thyroid problem | 14 | 12 | 85.7% | 2 | 14.3% |
| Other | 24 | 22 | 91.7% | 2 | 8.3% |

A. Reasons for the efficiency :

   a) Among the group with efficiency, more than 83 % both slap and pull.

b) b. Among the group with efficiency, more than 91 % insist on PL for more than1month.
c) c. Among the group with efficiency, more than 91 % slap and pull for a total hours more than 5.

B. Reasons for the inefficiency :

a) Short duration for PL, almost all within 1 month.
b) Short time for each Paida or Lajin, mostly less than 30 minutes.
c) c. The total time of the practice is mostly less than 1 hour.
d) d. Mere Paida or Lajin, without combining the two.
e) e. Do not acquire the method of PL in place and lack the theoretical learning.

**Conclusion:**

The effective rate is more than 80% for heart disease, diabetes, cervical spondylosis, periarthritis of shoulder and other 18 diseases, and the highest effective rate can reach 100%. Meanwhile, the longer the duration of PL, the better the effect.

## 4. Relation between the duration of PL and efficiency

We have divided into the following seven categories roughly:

Relation between the duration of PL and efficiency

| Duration with PL | Number of people | Only Lajin | Only Paida | Both PL | Effective number | Effective percentage |
| --- | --- | --- | --- | --- | --- | --- |
| Within 1 month | 18 | 0 | 8 | 10 | 11 | 61% |
| 1 to 3 months | 10 | 1 | 4 | 5 | 9 | 90% |
| 3 to 6 months | 11 | 1 | 1 | 9 | 11 | 100% |
| 6 to 12 | 15 | 1 | 1 | 13 | 14 | 93% |

| | | | | | | |
|---|---|---|---|---|---|---|
| months | | | | | | |
| 1 to 2 years | 36 | 2 | 2 | 32 | 36 | 100% |
| 2 to 5 years | 27 | 1 | 2 | 24 | 27 | 100% |
| 5 years and above | 20 | 0 | 2 | 18 | 20 | 100% |

**Analysis and conclusion:**

The efficiency is 61% for those insist on PL within 1 month, the efficiency can reach more than 90% basically for those who insist on it more than 1 month, while the efficiency can reach 100% basically for those who insist on it more than 3 months, including a netizen who insisted for a period between 6 and 12 months, but obtained no obvious effect, because the PL practice was in a weekly manner instead of daily, each time 30-60 minutes. Therefore, the longer the continuous duration of PL, the better the effect.

## 5. Relationship between PL and efficiency

Relationship between PL and efficiency

| Item | Number of people | Ratio | Efficiency |
|---|---|---|---|
| Only Lajin | 6 | 4.4% | 83% |
| Only Paida | 20 | 14.6% | 80% |
| Both PL | 111 | 81% | 94.6% |

81% of the 137 netizens both slap and pull, with the efficiency of 94.6%, 4.4% only pull, with the efficiency of 83%, and 14.6% only slap, with the efficiency of 80%. Therefore, the effect of combining the two is better the effect of one.

## 6. Improvement effect of pain by PL

With a full score of 10, 137 netizens scored the average pain of 6.27 points for the body pain maladies before PL, and 3.98 points after practicing PL. So we can see that PL can effectively reduce the pain.

To sum up,

1. PL is effective for heart disease, diabetes, cervical spondylosis, periarthritis of shoulder and other 18 diseases, and the effective rate is more than 80%.
2. Mere Paida or Lajin is effective, but it will more effective combining the two.
3. The longer the duration of PL, the better the effect. It is better that the practice can exceed more than 1 month.
4. PL can reduce the pain effectively.
5. Males are suggested to strengthen PL to improve their health

———Team of PL, on August 21, 2018

| Summary | Total number of people | Number of people with | Significant improvement | Improved the number of | Rate of improvement | Number of discontinued | Discontinuation rate |
|---|---|---|---|---|---|---|---|
| Total number of people | 61 | 57 | 93% | 4 | 7% | | |
| Hypertension and hypotension | 6 | 5 | 83% | 1 | 17% | 5 | 83% |
| Heart disease | 10 | 9 | 90% | 1 | 10% | 10 | 100% |
| Shoulder, neck and back pain | 9 | 9 | 100% | 0 | 0% | 9 | 100% |
| Arthropathy | 11 | 11 | 100% | 0 | 0% | 10 | 91% |
| Lumbocrural pain | 12 | 12 | 100% | 0 | 0% | 12 | 100% |
| Sub-health status | 1 | 1 | 100% | 0 | 0% | 0 | 0% |
| Astriction | 4 | 4 | 100% | 0 | 0% | 4 | 100% |
| Gynaopathy | 9 | 9 | 100% | 0 | 0% | 7 | 78% |
| Male diseases | 3 | 3 | 100% | 0 | 0% | 3 | 100% |
| Gastric disease | 11 | 9 | 82% | 2 | 18% | 9 | 82% |
| Poor sleep | 13 | 13 | 100% | 0 | 0% | 11 | 85% |
| Diabetes | 4 | 3 | 75% | 1 | 25% | 4 | 100% |

# Appendix 3: Statistics on the effect of PL self-healing method promoted by Boss Cao

There are the statistics of the self-healing effectiveness method promoted by the Chongqing businessman Boss Cao, who had promoted PL to over several thousands people, which is only a small part of the statistics. It was not found that those who insist on PL have not been effective. Is there a disadvantage to a good method? Of course, it is positive! The biggest disadvantage is the better effectiveness! The good effectiveness is incredible!

**Summary of self-healing statistics:**

1. Among the students in the statistics, more than 94% of hypertension, heart disease, diabetes, shoulder, neck, and back disease, lumbocrural pain, joint disease and major diseases are effective.
2. In the statistics, a total of 61 people insisted on PL, among which 93% of them improved their health and 7% of them improved their health significantly.
3. More than 85% of students who had previously taken medication stopped taking it.

# Appendix 4: The statistics of 200 documented cases were promoted by Boss Cao

1. The male-female ratio in the 200 cases with effectiveness is 47:53.
2. Among the 200 cases with effectiveness, people over 40 years old were accounted for 82% of cases with age records, which indicated that the middle-aged people pay the great important attention to the maintenance of body.
3. Names of the diseases involved in 200 cases were included: cold, astriction, insomnia, frozen shoulder, lumbago, cervical pain, stroke sequelae, depression, headache, sciatica, cough, loose stool, lumbar disc herniation, dizziness, gastrointestinal disease, tinnitus, diabetes, knee pain, no squat legs, thirst, Dowager's Hump, surgical sequelae, sub-health status, heat stroke, hypertension, chest tightness, hyperthyroidism, hand numbness, palm itching, cardiovascular and cerebrovascular diseases, kidney disease, ankle swelling, prostatitis hyperplasia, rheumatoid, lung cancer, synovitis, tenosynovitis, lumbocrural pain, facial paralysis, lumbar sprain, psoriasis, oral ulcers, left chest pain, left face pain, vertigo, prostatic hypertrophy, obesity, bitter mouth, drunkenness, dry mouth, hyperlipidemia, aphonia, butterfly sleeve, Parkinson's syndrome, heel tendonitis, tendon adhesions, left lower extremity arterial stasis, eczema, cystitis, hematuria, varicose veins, acne, seborrheic dermatitis, fainting, infertility, sleep apnea syndrome, hemorrhoids, stiff neck, cataracts, floaters, pneumonia, thyroid nodules, oral ulcers, sequelae of gas poisoning, gout, lumbar muscle strain, stomach swelling, crying and other 78 diseases, with the 100% effective rate, among which the Top 8 diseases are shown as below:

| Name of disease | Number of people | Number of people with effectiveness | Rate of effectiveness |
| --- | --- | --- | --- |
| | | | |

| | | | |
|---|---|---|---|
| Arthralgia | 101 | 101 | 100% |
| Gastrointestinal disease | 69 | 69 | 100% |
| Insomnia | 59 | 59 | 100% |
| Heart disease | 22 | 22 | 100% |
| Hypertension | 19 | 19 | 100% |
| Dizzy | 14 | 14 | 100% |
| Cold cough | 12 | 12 | 100% |
| Diabetes | 10 | 10 | 100% |

The largest number of diseases in the same individual was eight diseases.

4. Because Paida activities were held in Beibei Park all year round, where the Paida fellows had mastered the skillful and penetrating techniques, the intensity was many times greater than that of individuals at home. Therefore, there was also strong HC, including bruise, pain, crying, sweating, dizziness, palpitations and other reactions. It demonstrated that the Paida fellows did have meridian blockage as well as heart disease.

# Appendix 5: Statistical results of Zhang Yumei PL Health Club in Huizhou, guangdong

Since January 2015, a total of 143 registered clients at my Health Club had been registered for conditioning, of which the male-female ratio is 1:2.

Among the 143 people, a total of 143 people involved 83 diseases, including colds, astriction, insomnia, frozen shoulder, lumbago, cervical pain, stroke sequelae, depression, headache, sciatica, cough, lumbar disc herniation, dizziness, gout, stomach disease, tinnitus, diabetes, sub-health status, hypertension, heart disease, uterine fibroids, breast hyperplasia, gynaopathy, dysmenorrhea, thyroid nodules, menstrual irregularities, knee pain, cramps, rhinitis, pharyngitis, sprains, hyperlipidemia, high cholesterol, rheumatism, hand pain, foot pain, varicose veins, hyperthyroidism, uremia, chest pain, toothache, acne, itchy skin, lung cancer, back pain, stomach pain, nail fungus, endometriosis, ovarian cysts, bladder cancer, hepatitis B, hypotension, chest tightness, bloating, body cold, bone hyperplasia, osteoporosis, beriberi, anemia, emphysema, myocardial ischemia, bronchitis, myocardial infarction, fever, eczema, skin diseases, endocrine disorders, small intestinal stromal tumors, oral ulcers, ankylosing spondylitis, myocardial ischemia, chocolate cyst, acute myelitis, lymphoma, bile duct stones, gallbladder polyps, prostate enlargement, polycystic liver, polycystic kidney, prostatic enlargement, amenorrhea, breast cancer, lipoma and others, with an effective rate of 100%. Among them, the top 8 conditions are:

| Name of the disease | Number of sick people | Number of people with effective improvement | Effective rate |
|---|---|---|---|
| Lumbago | 20 | 20 | 100% |
| Sub-health status | 19 | 19 | 100% |
| Scapulohumeral periarthritis | 17 | 17 | 100% |

| | | | |
|---|---|---|---|
| Insomnia | 12 | 12 | 100% |
| Hypertension | 12 | 12 | 100% |
| Heart disease | 11 | 11 | 100% |
| Cervical spondylosis | 11 | 11 | 100% |
| Uterine fibroids | 11 | 11 | 100% |

There are 10 types of diseases that suffer from the most individual diseases. The common symptoms of HC are pain, bruise, nausea, vomiting, bloody urine, black urine, hiccups, cold sweat, and others.

Only 5 people registered to take the drug, of which 4 of them stopped taking the drug and 1 of them reduced the drug.

# Appendix 6: Investigation Report of PL by Hebei Zhao Ruihua

The self-healing method of PL is a non-medical method, without any drug administration, which can activate the Qi and blood of body, to enhance self-healing power, achieve the purpose of adjusting the body, improve the various discomforts, and regain health. This method is easy to learn, real and effective. In the spring of 2013, I was introduced to this method. While conditioning his body step by step, he also began to promote it to friends around him. We have organized many mutual-Paida events, and more and more people have accepted this method and benefited more and more. In the process of promoting it, I found that although the self-healing method has benefited tens of millions of people in recent years and has spread to more than 50 countries, there are still many people who have never heard of it, and most people do not understand this method, and deny its efficacy based on subjective speculation. What is the effect of the self-healing method of PL? From April to August 2018, I spent five months investigating the condition of 30 Paida fellows who persisted on before and after PL.

There are the results of my survey:

| NO. | | Total number of | People with the | Rate of improvement | Number of people with | Number of people with drug reduction | Rate of drug reduction |
|---|---|---|---|---|---|---|---|
| NO. | Total number of people | 30 | 30 | 100% | 28 | 2 | 6.7% |
| 1 | Heart disease | 5 | 5 | 100% | 5 | | |
| 2 | Hypertension | 2 | 2 | 100% | 2 | | |
| 3 | Diabetes | 3 | 3 | 100% | 1 | 2 | 67% |
| 4 | Shoulder, neck and back pain | 7 | 7 | 100% | 4 | Three of them were not on medication | |
| 5 | Lumbocrural pain | 11 | 11 | 100% | 11 | | |
| 6 | Dermatosis | 3 | 3 | 100% | 3 | | |

| 7 | Gastroenterology | 7 | 7 | 100% | 7 | |
|---|---|---|---|---|---|---|
| 8 | Gynaopathy | 4 | 4 | 100% | | |
| 9 | Cough | 2 | 2 | 100% | 2 | |
| 10 | Prostate | 3 | 3 | 100% | | |
| 11 | Hemorrhoids | 1 | 1 | 100% | 1 | |
| 12 | Rhinitis | 2 | 2 | 100% | 2 | |
| 13 | Floaters | 1 | 1 | 100% | | |
| 14 | Get up at night to urinate | 6 | 6 | 100% | | |
| 15 | Dizziness and headache | 2 | 2 | 100% | 2 | |
| 16 | Toothache | 1 | 1 | 100% | 1 | |
| 17 | cosmetology and slimming | 9 | 9 | 100% | | |
| 18 | Ankylosing spondylitis | 2 | 2 | 100% | 1 | One of them was not on medication |
| 19 | Oral ulcer | 1 | 1 | 100% | 1 | |
| 20 | Sleep problems | 4 | 4 | 100% | 4 | |
| 21 | Urethritis | 3 | 3 | 100% | 3 | |
| 22 | Sub-health status | 3 | 3 | 100% | | |

## I. Basic situation

Among the 30 respondents, there were people from thirty years old to seventy years old, from the young to the old, which covered different age groups. Among them, 23 respondents were women, accounting for 76.7%, and 7 respondents were men, accounting for 23.3%. Their diseases covered 22 types, including diseases, including heart disease, hyperglycemia, diabetes, lumbocrural pain and other. Except for gynecology, prostate disease, floaters, getting up at night to urinate, cosmetology and slimming, and sub-health status, all of which have not been used, the rest of the drug Paida fellows have stopped or reduced their medication. Among them, 28 people stopped taking drugs, accounting for 93.3%, and 2 people reduced drugs, accounting for

6.7%. The improvement rate of hypertension, heart disease, diabetes, shoulder and neck pain, lumbocrural pain, gastroenterology, prostate disease, getting up at night and other major conditions to urinate had reached 100%.

## II. Results of survey

1. PL had a good effectiveness on the specific common pains. Among 30 respondents, 11 respondents had lumbocrural pain, accounting for 36.7%; 7 respondents had shoulder, neck and back pain, accounting for 23.3%, who took the various painkillers before PL. Moreover, some respondents were treated with acupuncture, small-needle-scalpel and other traditional Chinese medicine methods before PL. All of them had stopped drugs after PL, with 100% self-healing effect.
2. PL had a significant effect on cosmetology and slimming. Without exception, the complexion of all surveyed Paida fellows had changed greatly after PL than before, the weight of the fat people had decreased after PL. Moreover, two people who showed the thin body shape in the past had increased their weight significantly.
3. PL can act in the treatment and regulation of the heart mainly. The process of PL is inseparable from the role of mental force, the pain of PL is also directed to the heart. If you can actively accept the pain of PL, the self-healing effect of the body can be better, whose body and mind is harmonious, accompanied with the cheerful mood. It can also be seen from the change in the mentality of the survey subjects that PL can heal the body disease as well as the heart disease, to improve the mental strength. Among the 30 Paida fellows surveyed, their personalities generally changed from negative introverts to optimistic and cheerful mood after PL.
4. The self-healing method of PL is simple, safe and effective. The Paida fellows who insist on PL are not professional medical professional. However, they can quickly learn to PL and heal their own diseases by the

method. From the common lumbocrural pain, neck and shoulder pain to ankylosing spondylitis, most diseases classified by modern medicine are almost self-healed. The unexplained sub-health status classified by the modern medicine also has better results. Moreover, the method is safe without any danger.
5. The self-healing method of PL has low cost and environmental protection. Most of 30 Paida fellows surveyed insisted on PL every day, except for 2 people who reduced their medication, all their bodies were better after stopping taking the drug, compared with the period when they took the drug. From the economic point of view, it can save a lot of medical expenses for the family. Besides, it can also reduce the pollution of drugs and equipment to the body and nature, to avoid the waste of resources and energy. From the perspective of a country, it can save a lot of medical expenses. Moreover, it can also ease the tension between doctors and patients and reduce the pollution of the whole nature. It can truly benefit the country, the people, and mankind.

## III. The issues that shall notice

1. PL is not effective for everyone. The main difference between the self-healing method and the medical method is the own diligently intention. Therefore, people who do not believe PL or do not start PL will not have an effectiveness. Some of the 30 respondents without the obvious effect at first. The strength of PL was reduced for some improved symptoms, the physical condition repeats itself repeatedly. However, they eventually persisted PL. Whether it is an emergency or chronic disease, it will be effective if you insist on PL. If you will be suspicious of PL, without the strong execution, the effect would be greatly reduced.
2. 2. The self-healing method of PL cannot be viewed with the concept of Western medicine. PL is fundamentally different from Western medicine, so that you cannot look at the various phenomena by the viewpoint of Western medicine that occurs during PL. Western medicine is

symptomatic treatment, for which the drugs and surgeries often suppress symptoms. The lesions often can be revealed by PL. Therefore, it will be various uncomfortable symptoms during PL. In fact, the known and unknown diseases can be revealed, they can be gradually resolved. From the viewpoint of Western medicine, it is a phenomenon of aggravation of symptoms.
3. Individual PL is not as good as the collective PL. Among the survey subjects, many people often participate in Mutual-Paida activities, compared to their own individual Paida, the fellows with the frequent Mutual-Paida have stronger mental strength and better self-healing effect.
4. It is better to combine PL. Some respondents are fond of Paida, and some respondents focus on Lajin. Paida will work better combined with Lajin. The individual Paida or Lajin will affect the effect of PL.

## IV. Conclusion

Although the self-healing method of PL is not a medical act, everyone can do PL, if you do it wholeheartedly, the effect will exceed the current traditional Chinese medicine and Western medicine. It is simple to learn and easy to popularize. There is natural, simple, and effective whole process, which can be diagnosed and treated, as well as disease prevention and fitness. Moreover, it is low cost and safe without any side effects, which is suitable for the large-scale promotion in humans.

# Appendix 7: Statistics on the effectiveness of the self-healing method of PL by Hubei Green Walnut

Green Walnut, served as a bank clerk, promoted the result of PL: self-healing efficiency was 100%, it was similar to the statistical results of Boss Cao. Is there anything that doesn't work well? Certainly! The effectiveness of the following categories of people is not obvious.

1. People who want to heal a bunch of physical diseases and only have patience for one day;
2. People who want to find a divine doctor to heal you and do not want to change themselves;
3. People already have a good regimen;
4. People who do not want to spend 1 hour a day to maintain their bodies;
5. People who go fishing for three days and dry their nets for two days.

|  | Total number of | Number of people | Significant improvement | Number of people | Rate of improvement |
|---|---|---|---|---|---|
| Overall symptom | 45 | 45 | 100% | 0 | 0% |
| Hypertension/hypotension | 3 | 3 | 100% | 0 | 0% |
| Heart Diseases | 5 | 5 | 100% | 0 | 0% |
| Shoulder, neck and back pain | 10 | 10 | 100% | 0 | 0% |
| Arthropathy | 4 | 4 | 100% | 0 | 0% |
| Lumbocrural pain | 12 | 12 | 100% | 0 | 0% |
| Sub-health status | 7 | 7 | 100% | 0 | 0% |
| Astriction | 2 | 2 | 100% | 0 | 0% |
| Gynaopathy | 7 | 7 | 100% | 0 | 0% |
| Male diseases | 0 | 0 | 0% | 0 | 0% |

| | | | | | |
|---|---|---|---|---|---|
| Gastric disease | 4 | 4 | 100% | 0 | 0% |
| Poor sleep quality | 6 | 6 | 100% | 0 | 0% |
| Diabetes | 1 | 1 | 100% | 0 | 0% |

**Summary of self-healing statistics:**

1. Among the students in the statistics, it is 100% effective to the students with hypertension, heart disease, diabetes, shoulder, neck and back disease, lumbocrural pain, joint disease and other major diseases.
2. According to the statistics, 45 people persisting in PL, whose health improved significantly, accounting for 100%.

# Appendix 8: Shandong Yimu (retired driver) spread the effect of PL statistical table

This is the data of retired old driver Yimu promoting the statistics of PL. Although it is several data, it is convincing. For the privacy, the real name is replaced by a number.

| Number of Name | Duration of PL | Whether it has an effect | Whether to reduce the drug and stop the drug | Medical costs reduced or not |
|---|---|---|---|---|
| 001 | Two and a half year | Effective | Drug withdrawal | No medical cost |
| 002 | Two and a half year | Effective | Drug withdrawal | No medical cost |
| 003 | More than 2 years | Effective | Drug withdrawal | No medical cost |
| 004 | More than 2 years | Effective | Drug withdrawal | No medical cost |
| 005 | More than 2 years | Effective | Drug reduction | Reduce medical cost |
| 006 | More than 1 year | Effective | Drug reduction | Reduce medical cost |
| 007 | More than 1 year | Effective | Drug reduction | Reduce medical cost |
| 008 | More than 1 year | Effective | Drug withdrawal | No medical cost |
| 009 | More than 1 year | Effective | Drug withdrawal | No medical cost |
| 010 | 1 year | Effective | Drug reduction | Reduce medical cost |
| 011 | 1 year | Effective | Drug withdrawal | Reduce medical cost |
| 012 | 1 year | Effective | Drug reduction | Reduce medical cost |
| 013 | 1 year | Effective | Drug reduction | Reduce medical cost |
| 014 | 1 year | Effective | Drug | No medical |

| | | | withdrawal | cost |
|---|---|---|---|---|
| 015 | 1 year | Effective | Drug withdrawal | No medical cost |

**Summary of self-healing statistics:**

1. A total of 15 practitioners have persisted with PL for at least a year, with 100% effectiveness.
2. A total of 60% students who had previously taken the drug stopped taking the drug, 40% of them reduced the dose.
3. In conclusion, 53.3% of people had no medical cost, 46.7% of them reduced the medical costs.

If everyone can insist on PL to heal themselves, the family's medical expenses will be greatly reduced, for which it can greatly save the country's expenses. Moreover, it is also environmentally friendly!

www.ingramcontent.com/pod-product-compliance
Lightning Source LLC
Chambersburg PA
CBHW071205240526
45470CB00018B/1479